To my
Love!

Forever,
Linda

Menopause: Just The Facts, Ma'am!

by
Neil C. Boland and Linda LaVelle

Bloomington, IN Milton Keynes, UK

authorHOUSE®

AuthorHouse™
1663 Liberty Drive, Suite 200
Bloomington, IN 47403
www.authorhouse.com
Phone: 1-800-839-8640

AuthorHouse™ UK Ltd.
500 Avebury Boulevard
Central Milton Keynes, MK9 2BE
www.authorhouse.co.uk
Phone: 08001974150

First published by AuthorHouse 9/13/2006

ISBN: 1-4259-5532-0 (sc)
ISBN: 1-4259-5531-2 (dj)

Printed in the United States of America
Bloomington, Indiana

This book is printed on acid-free paper.

Library of Congress Control Number: 2006907418

Acknowledgments

The authors wish to express our heartfelt appreciation and a special "Thank You" to a group of individuals without whose help this book would not be a success! We simply could not have done this without you.

To Bob Klunk for Cover Artwork : Klunkart@aol.com,
To Leslie Driver for Cartoon Work: Lesleyeld@aol.com,
To Sabrina Glover forArtistry: Sabrina@blackravendesigns.com
To Jonathan Boland and Jay Petersen for IT Management,
To Rick Petelinkar for helping us choose Author House,
To Bob Dobens for Photographic Expertise,
To Lisa Vinson for Salon Management,
To The Everett Collection, Inc., in New York City for their gracious licensed permission to use original photography from the timeless 1939 movie "The Wizard of Oz"
www.everettcollection.com,
as well as to the wonderful professional publishers of
www.AuthorHouse.com

ea ea ea

<u>Menopause, Just The Facts, Ma'am!</u>

You may Email, visit the authors, or order online additional copies of this book at the Book's Official Website: <u>www.justthefactsmaam.net</u>.

Linda Lavelle: <u>MenopauseJTFM@bellsouth.net</u>
Dr. Neil C. Boland: <u>DrBoland@justthefactsmaam.net</u>

About The Authors

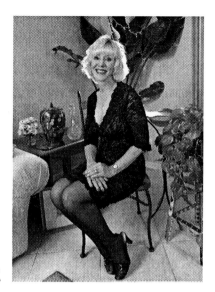

Linda LaVelle A.T.I.E., I.T.E.C.

LINDA LAVELLE began her 35 year career in aesthetics in the early 1970s. During that time, she studied under the most renown names in cosmetics and skin care worldwide, including Christine Valmy of New York, Marvin Westmore in California, Joel Gerson "Master of Skin Care Education", Martin Jans in Holland, and Jean D'Estrees of Paris, France.

Linda holds dozens of certifications in all areas of cosmetics, skin care, and hair care. Most recently, she earned her Diploma in Beauty Specialty from the International Therapy Examination Council (ITEC). Recognized worldwide in 19 countries, ITEC is the largest international examination board offering the highest professional esthetic diplomas possible. She is one of a handful of aesthetists in the state of Florida who is board certified and has been awarded ITEC accreditation.

Linda has worked as a make-up artist and skin care technician for Syd Simons Salon & Studio and Playboy International prior to opening Linda LaVelle's Spa d'Esthetiques in 1983. The spa was recognized as "Day Spa of the Year for the Treasure Coast" in 2004 and Linda was named the 2004 "Republican Business Woman of the Year" for the state of Florida.

While running her very successful spa in Stuart, Florida, Linda continues her education to address the skin care needs in the medical community. Working in conjunction with physicians, Linda provides pre and post operative skin care for plastic surgery patients with special chemical peels and Microdermabrasion, as well as facial lymphatic and esthetic drainage.

Just the Facts Ma'am, is Linda's First Book. Through it, she hopes to continue her work helping women to live life the fullest and enjoy the skin they're in. Linda lives in Stuart, Florida with her husband Bobby P., and her son, Sean.

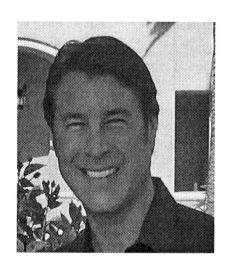

About The Authors

Neil C. Boland, M.D. F.A.C.O.G.

DR. NEIL C. BOLAND, M.D., F.A.C.O.G. received his B.S. degree Magna Cum Laude With Honors from Florida State University in 1973 in Biological Science.   In 1977, he received his M.D. degree from the Emory University School of Medicine in Atlanta, Georgia. He did his internship and residency training in Gynecology and Obstetrics at the Emory University Affiliated Hospitals, completing his training there in 1981. Subsequently, he became Board-Certified in the field of Ob/Gyn in 1983, and voluntarily recertified in 1994 by the American Board of Ob/Gyn. He has since been in the private practice in the Stuart, Florida area, having delivered over 5,000 babies, recently specializing in the relatively new field of Menopausal Medicine.

Dr. Boland has been extremely active in clinical research, having participated in over 60 collaborative research projects since 1992 in the fields of gynecologic oncology, endocrinology, osteoporosis, female sexual dysfunction, and nicotine addiction.   In 1981, he was the first researcher in history to prove nicotine does indeed cross the human placental barrier into the fetus during pregnancy in smoking mothers with multiple detrimental effects. He is an Affiliate Faculty Member of the H. Lee Mofitt Cancer and Research Institute, University of South Florida, in Tampa.

He has been an Obstetrical Consultant to NASA (National Aeronautics and Space Administration) in Cape Canaveral, Florida as a physician to astronauts and their families. Castle-Connolly Medical, Ltd. Of New York has named him one of the "Best Doctors in Florida", and he was recently honored for inclusion in the "Guide to America's Top Obstetricians and Gynecologists" (2004-2005 edition) by the Consumer's Research Council of America.

In 2002, Dr. Boland became credentialed by the North American Menopause Society as a Certified Menopausal Practitioner. In 2004, he helped co-found Advanced Laser Therapy, a new company dedicated to the use of lasers in the treatment of nicotine addiction and other disorders. He is an institutional review board consultant in this field to the U.S. Food and Drug Administration. As a professional tenor saxophonist, he started his own rock and roll band in 1999, the "Jazzernauts Rock and Soul Revue", which today are known as "The Rhythm Doctors". Hobbies of sailing, fishing, and strength conditioning help him keep perspective as well.

Dedications

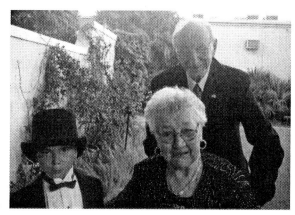

This book is dedicated to Aunt El, Bobby, and Sean whom I love with all of my heart and soul!   To Aunt El, thank you for your faith, your strength, and the love you gave me during my childhood and adult years. To Bobby, thank you for loving me, and pushing me into anger so that I could write this book with courage and determination. To my son Sean, thank you for loving me the way a mommy should be loved, and accepting me the way I am! I love you dearly!

Linda Lavelle, A.T.I.E., I.T.E.C.
July 8, 2006

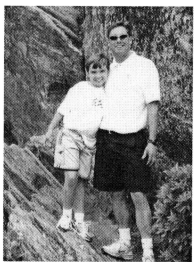

Menopause and Face Lift Advice:

The face gets them to bed. The breasts keep them in bed…..and don't worry about the damn tummy, who cares? You got him!
Joan Rivers

Live a Life of Happiness~

Happiness cannot come from without. It must come from within. It is not what we see and touch or that which others do for us which makes us happy; it is that which we think and feel and do, first for the other fellow and then for ourselves.
Helen Keller

Carry These Gifts Of The Heart~

Trust….That whatever happens, there is someone who will understand. Honesty…..The feeling that you never need to hold back. Peace…..In being accepted for who you really are. Beauty….in outlook more than appearance. Freedom…..To be yourself, to change and to grow. Joy…...In every day, in every memory, and in your hopes for the future. Love…… To last a lifetime, and perhaps beyond.
D.L. Riepl

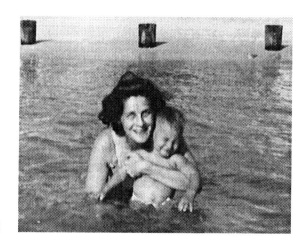

Dedications

This book is dedicated to my mother, Louise Boland Harrison, whom I dearly love. Here we are swimming together in 1953. She was a Georgia school teacher for many years, teaching me to read and write at an early age. She provided me with a solid academic foundation for a future career in medicine and research. Her teachings and guidance continue to influence thousands of Americans today.

I also wish to dedicate this book to the heroic men and women of the FDNY and the 911 tragedy, and our incredibly brave U.S. troops serving in Iraq and Afghanistan.
Neil C. Boland, M.D., F.A.C.O.G.
June 28, 2006

The society of women is the foundation of good manners.
Johann Wolfgang von Goethe, Die Wahlverwandtschaften

O Woman, you are not merely the handiwork of God, but also of men; these are ever endowing you with beauty from their own hearts. . . . You are one-half woman and one-half dream.
Rabindranath Tagore, Gardener

A group of recognizably high-powered media women on the shady side of forty were spaced around the table between their husbands and lovers at a Washington dinner party when a single sentence shattered their well-groomed calm. It came out of the mouth of the stunning network newswoman who ordinarily speaks in ninety-second bursts of inside-the-Beltway shorthand.

"Okay, there are only two subjects worth talking about--menopause and face-lifts." It was as though a nine-hundred-pound gorilla had just jumped up on the table.

Gail Sheehy - The Silent Passage

Foreword

By Linda La Velle, A.T.I.E., I.T.E.C.

Menopause is not an easy thing to write about. Most women are afraid to talk about it, as they fear that no one else is like them in their thoughts and feelings. Well, you are!!

Ever thought about driving the car into a pole at night because you are so angry? How about not wanting to get up in the morning because you are very depressed? Better yet, waking up and finding a person who you do not know jumping down the throats of your loved one or your co-workers. I can vividly remember my mother sitting at the kitchen table crying her eyes out, and wondering why she just had painted a white couch in the living room black!

These incidents are very real and I personally have experienced some of them in perimenopause and the onset of it. The night sweats and hot flashes are a common thing that we think we must endure, and we go on accepting it, trying to find a natural solution to solve some of our problems. For most women, this natural solution does not work. I was one of them! For one year, I struggled with Gingko Biloba for forgetfulness, Black Cohosh, yam, and soy protein along with a myriad of vitamins to supplement my hormone losses. I even tried natural progesterone cream and testosterone cream from my local Health Food Store. I would rub them on my legs and arms faithfully with no change in my hot flashes or night sweats. The worst thing was my forgetfulness, as here I am running a Day Spa and Salon and I can't get from my retail area to my office and remember what I am doing there!

My skin was getting drier. I was getting bitchier and my sex life was in a total disaster! I found that I had no desire for sex, and I had a wonderful husband lying next to me wondering why I am not sexually excited by him?

It started five years previously, and perimenopause was at it's onset. I went to my Gynecologist and he tried everything to help me. This included estrogen during my periods to calm me down, vitamin B complex, and also wanted to put me on birth control pills monthly. I was afraid to go back on the birth control pills because I had taken them for almost 20 years and was afraid of getting cancer from the hormone therapy. I tried the natural approach with vitamin therapy and natural teas to keep me from waking up in the middle of the night. I worked out regularly which really helped my serotonin level, but I was still getting angry or depressed before my periods.

I can honestly say that I was afraid to tell my Gynecologist my feelings for fear that he would put me on some psychotic drug to calm me down or change my moods and I was convinced that this abnormal behavior was due to my hormones fluctuating greatly. So, I tried to live with them and accept the person that was inside of me. The person inside of me was not sane all of the time and my calm demeanor was slowly disappearing. I was getting very frustrated.

I remember one incident that literally drove me to my Gynecologist. I went away for a week with my husband up to the North Carolina mountains and we stayed at a beautiful Bed and Breakfast overlooking the Blue Ridge Parkway. It was the ultimate view and the most relaxing thing that you could imagine. Somehow, I managed to start a huge fight over what we would have for dinner and I walked out the door. Now mind you, this was in the heart of the mountains. I walked down to a nearby town to calm down. There was an old hotel at the bottom of the ridge. I walked up to the hotel's porch and sat in a rocking chair to clear my head. Before I knew it, it was dark and I did not know what road to take to find the place we were staying. I walked up two different roads followed by night flies trying to find my cabin. After a few wrong turns, the cabin turned up! When I walked into the cabin, I asked my husband why he didn't search for me. He responded, "You were angry as all hell and I thought you took the car, so I figured I'd let you calm down. We made up of course. Then I realized I had lost part of my sanity, plus my thinking ability was becoming distorted and my memory loss was increasing.

I can remember vividly wanting to go to Home Depot one morning and driving by it as my son says "Mom, you just drove by Home Depot"! That was the last straw. I decided to take hold of my life and see my Gynecologist again. He then suggested I do Balloon Ablation surgery to put me right into menopause as my periods were out of control and my mind was right there with it as well.

This surgery at the time was fairly new, but it worked beautifully. My periods stopped instantly and I found a new life coming on my hormones were at a new level. I was looking for my former self, once again.

Slowly a new woman emerged. One without any hormones at all. My hot flashes increased by twenty a day. My night sweats were at 2 A.M.. I would rip my night gown off, wait a few minutes and then put it back on as I got chilled. After a couple of night sweats, you learn to go to bed naked and you leave your night gown by the side of the bed just in case you get cold. Your personal life, especially with your husband becomes intolerable as he knows not what to do except to put his golf cap on, wear socks to bed and sleep in his long johns as the temperature in the house must be set as frigid as the North Pole.

Again, I took a trek to the gynecologist with my hormone ups and downs. This time I was near tears, I said "Doctor, you have to help me control these imbalances and I can no longer take it!" That is when he stepped in and explained why I was having all of these problems. You see, a woman's hormone imbalance can be a myriad of 25 things going wrong in your body. When your ovaries are dead, no hormones are being pumped into your system, so it is up to the doctor to try and figure out what hormones you are lacking and believe me, this does take some time.

You cannot fill a hormone concoction for everyone and expect it to fit. You have to work with each patient's hormone problems and dissect what would work best with their imbalance.

This is why my gynecologist and I decided to write this book. Hopefully our anger and frustration with hormone problems can make others understand what menopause is really about!

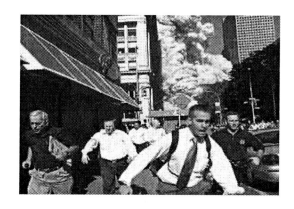

Foreword

By Neil C. Boland, M.D., F.A.C.O.G.

On September 11, 2001, a group of foreign national terrorists known as Al-Quaeda hijacked and then piloted two jet airliners into the World Trade Center in Manhattan. Two other jets crashed that day, causing well over 3,000 citizen casualties. As Americans, our daily lives have been forever changed...... and in our lifetime, we will somehow never feel exactly as secure as we did before 911. In short, this was truly a life changing event for all of us.

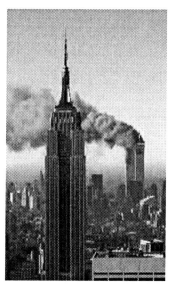

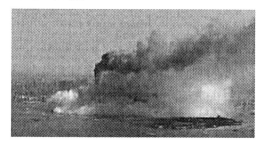

We now realize that 911 for the menopausal and peri-menopausal woman did not occur until about ten months later. On that date, July 22, 2002, a massive landmark study called The Womens Health Initiative (WHI) was published in the Journal Of The American Medical Association (JAMA). This well done prospective controlled multicenter medical study involved the use of two specific types of oral combination hormonal therapy (HT), following over 161,000 patients over eight years.

The WHI study involved the study of possible increased or decreased risks in these patients on HT relative to breast cancer, heart attack, stroke, thromboembolism (blood clot) complications, colon cancer, and hip fracture, as well as multiple other disease states. It attempted to quantify these risks, with some risks being statistically significant, and some not significant. This data was presented in a purely scholarly and scientific fashion, clearly with little peer review. There were no verifiable recommendations for action attached at that time. Prior to its publication, women were prescribed HT with much more liberal indications, such as hot flashes, night sweats, vaginal atrophy, osteoporosis, and even with the off label indications of prevention of cardiovascular disease and dementia.

It is not generally well known that the American media have access to medical journal information at least a week in advance of the public, including physicians. The print and television media pounced on the WHI Study and electrified the public with pure science, opportunistically drawing their own conclusions, with a "See, I-Told-You-So-Attitude". Well, if da glove don't fit, you must blame, not acquit. It was as if the press itself became the sheriff's officer, baliff, judge, and jury for HT just because they had actually read the study. In horror and long painful anticipation, other U.S. physicians, including internists, family doctors, endocrinologists, cardiologists, oncologists, and Ob/Gyns, had to wait almost a week before the study was even published on the Internet, just to read this complex study.

No buildings collapsed on July 22, 2002. No one died in an airplane . No plume of white smoke or mushroom cloud emanated from the ivory towers of academia. No danger or destruction at the Pentagon or White House. What was heard instead that day was the deafening cacophonous *clanking of millions of trash cans* across the world, as menopausal women tossed their various medications of HT into the garbage.

It had to be really detrimental to their health, or the media wouldn't be making such a big deal out of this, would they? Toss it first, and ask questions later. I mean really.... What were their physicians thinking in prescribing this stuff? How could the number one prescribed medicine in world history for over forty years be so bad?

How could so many health care professionals be so wrong simultaneously? Physicians' phones rang off the hook. A totally panic-striken and confused public tried to contact an exhausted medical profession that had been set up perfectly for failure and given no advance information. The Titanic then began to sink as the health care system collapsed into chaotic disarray.

Fortunately, over the next several months and years, scientific rationality slowly began to emerge in the health care support system of menopausal women of America. Both physicians and patients began to discover why hormonal therapy was necessary for some patients and superfluous for others. Feeling absolutely miserable, millions of depressed, anxious, and sleep-deprived patients waving hand fans began to descend on doctor consultation rooms. An earnest reevaluation of medication pros and cons, risk and benefits, side effects, and alternatives, relative to the WHI was initiated. Frank discussion, calmness, and careful deliberate thought was used in the reevaluation of these women. Others have waited their turn.

These patients have seemed to fall into four general categories. After physician evaluation, some patients were taken off HT for good and are doing fine. The WHI Study has helped us all refocus on risk and benefits of hormonal replacement.

A second group have gone back on HT, felt great, and reverted back to their old selves. Their spouses, families, and co-workers have all breathed a huge sigh of relief.

A third group headed for the Internet to find their own medical nirvana, many being financially victimized by non-prescription "natural" creams and other remedies, about which the safety and effectiveness have never been proven scientifically, because they have never received F.D.A. approval. Unfortunately, a lot of them (about 18%) received "placebo relief", and could have achieved the same effect by rubbing toothpaste on their arms at considerably less cost.

A fourth group of patients continues today to wander from doctor to chiropractor searching for a "magic bullet" potion that is 100% guaranteed safe, extensively tested on millions of patients, without any side effects whatsoever, 100% effective, biodegradable, is "natural", gives them a raging sex drive, and is not made by a pharmaceutical company which is inhumane to mice. These patients seem to be amazed that the other three groups of patients even exist.

Menopause, Just The Facts, Ma'am has been written for each individual menopausal or soon to be menopausal woman. The first wave of post-World War II Baby Boomers became menopausal several years ago. This is a very complex multidisciplinary subject, and new information, new treatments, and new pharmaceuticals are constantly evolving. Carefully digest the information in this book which has been formulated from multiple medical specialities. Use it to become as informed as possible, and then talk with your health care professional about any questions you may have. Pass this book along to a friend or relative.

We have written this book because of the INTENSE AND OVERWHELMING NATIONAL DEMAND in 2006 that women have for accurate, unbiased, and latest up-to-date information on menopause, which is concise and readable. Menopause is complex. The media are killing us with confusion because they are confused themselves. We have tried to put this book in as simple vocabulary as possible, and explain terms where necessary. Most importantly, we are *not here to sell you a product such as a progesterone cream out of the back of our automobiles or on the Internet which has never been studied as far as safety or effectiveness. We also do not sell exercise equipment. We have to be experts in hormonal therapy.*

Remember, if you do have your menopausal health, you have just about everything. A corollary is that if you have poor quality of life due to severe menopausal symptoms, the rest of life really doesn't really matter that much anyway.

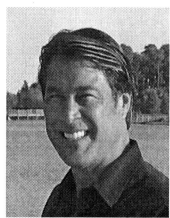

Table of Contents

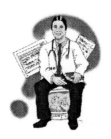

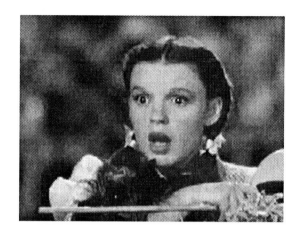

Chapter 1:

Menopause, Baby Boomers, The Internet, And The Rise of Medical Quackery: The Perfect Storm

By Neil C. Boland, M.D., F.A.C.O.G.

Houston, We Have A Problem!

The Internet, television, and the print media have done a woefully inadequate job in communicating our present understanding of the menopause to the vast majority of the female public. It often seems to me that new research findings presented to the general public as dogma has been already filtered by the media for maximum "shock value", because that is how the media derive maximum advertising dollar. Disappointingly, a lot of the information reaching the general public is actually written by non-physicians, trying to interpret scientifically complex data.

Even worse, publication and broadcast of this headline filtered information always occurs before over 99% of practicing physicians in America have even had an opportunity to review it. Press releases often occur before even the date of publication of data in scientific journals.

As such, an informationally hungry public is extremely vulnerable to misinterpreted and incorrect information.

Medicine tends to be complex, and is rarely definitive by being either black or white. The appropriate color is usually gray, with the unique need to be individualized for each patient. The words always and never are almost never appropriate in medicine. This makes our job, as your healthcare provider, much more difficult. Patients now frequently come to the office with preconceived biases and prejudices, which have originated from perhaps a well-meaning but misinformed fingernail technician.

In addition, in researching writing this book, I have discovered a pitiful lack of available general information about menopause available to women. The few books available to women are rarely written by authorities, but instead by individuals who either have an ax to grind with someone, or they have discovered a revolutionary new therapy, which of course, "naturally" allows them to profit by selling a proprietary "new" product or concept. Never mind that their new product has zero scientific credibility, because they know the public will buy it.

It is as if virtually all of our real pharmacologic research, perhaps involving some the most studied medications to mankind, are now somehow passé, irrelevant, and carcinogenic. Why? Because it pays (them) to say so. These purported new products seem to work about as well as a sugar pill (19%, or the so-called placebo effect) most the time. Totally confused and mystified, they then return to their physician for answers. Women are hungry.......hungry for valid informative answers to their questions. *Therein lies why writing a book of this magnitude is of such importance.*

Chances are excellent that on any given day that your doctor has already seen several patients that day that have stopped their hormonal therapy (HT) on their own. A lot of them are absolutely miserable, and felt much, much better taking their medication. They report they stopped because of "the cancer scare" or they "have heard horror stories" or their cousin's dog groomer "got breast cancer from that stuff". Their doctors then ask if they had received any communication from their offices to stop their medication, and patients report " no, not really". There are good reasons why they haven't.

Junk Science Leads to Junk Litigation

Even sadder now, the Florida television airwaves now boldly broadcast that such and such law firm now wants to talk with you...... but only if you have taken any estrogen product in the last sixty years and coincidentally were diagnosed with any form of breast cancer. YOU may be entitled to monetary damages! Never mind that one in eight women are diagnosed with breast cancer eventually anyway if they live to 110 whether they take hormones or not. (Similarly, eighty percent of men are diagnosed with prostate cancer by age 80.) Never mind that the published 2002 WHI Studies show only a tiny minimal breast cancer association, if any at all. Never mind that scientific cause and effect has never been proven. Never mind that followup WHI Studies with patients taking plain estrogen without progesterone show reduced rates of breast cancer compared with those patients taking no hormonal therapy.

Attorneys know all they have to do is create the illusion of MAYBE a cause and effect in front of a trial jury, and presto... Instant millionaires.....usually the attorney as well! Yep...Roll the dice. Connect the dots. Honey, we don't need to go to Vegas anymore. (They may not have to go to Vegas to gamble, but it's a sure bet their and everyone else's healthcare premiums will continue to escalate.)

Junk science (coupled with junk media broadcasting) can and will bamboozle society again! And who really pays the verdict? We all do!

Medical inflation is crippling America in the forms of higher insurance health insurance premiums for medical care. For example, your health care provider radiologist today will likely order many more screening mammographic extra views than they formerly did, as well as followup imaging studies. This leads to thousands of negative breast biopsies and needless patient anxiety. If he or she does not diagnose breast cancer every single time at its earliest possible *potential* appearance, a lawsuit will likely follow, even though mammography is *widely known to be only 80% accurate* as a limitation of the technology itself.

Eventually we will all end up paying higher homeowner insurance rates after Hurricanes Katrina, Rita, Wilma, and after HT lawsuits as well for breast cancer. We all pay for junk science, and it has to stop. In my opinion, the solution to this problem lies in a better educated public, removal of medical malpractice cases from the tort system instead to tribunals, better policing of the legal profession, and elimination of the lottery mentality. *Society as a whole will never be able to litigate itself into either prosperity or greatness.* Your physician is already policed and micromanaged far beyond what you may realize......hospital and peer review, insurance companies, Medicare auditing, state licensure boards, long before civil litigation aka so called "medical malpractice".

In some areas of the U.S. today, it is becoming impossible to even get a mammogram, with six month waits being reported. Why? What doctor would ever read a mammogram and dictate a report if it is it is only 80% accurate? Why is it in Florida some major metropolitan areas cannot even hire a radiologist to read mammograms for those doctors who retire? The answer is obvious.

To Take Or Not To Take HT- That Is The Question

It has to be explained that a percentage of some patients annually are indeed deliberately taken off HT by physicians because of the development of new diagnoses which do absolutely or relatively contraindicate therapy. An example of this would be development of a leg blood clot (called thrombophlebitis), ischemic colitis, breast cancer, or increased risk factors for cardiovascular disease. The medication should be stopped immediately if these conditions develop. These are the exceptions, not the rule, and will be individually addressed in later chapters.

Chances are also excellent your doctor does not have the luxury of endless time to explain to you in detail why going off HT might be a bad idea if for nothing else than quality of life (QOL) issues. Insurance companies and Medicare have consistently lowered reimbursements for office visit durations year after year for at least 13 of the last 14 years. There is barely enough time to cover routine screening checklists at your annual preventative office visit. We all know what happens when office overhead equals or exceeds reimbursement in the business world—look at Delta or Northwest Airlines. They go bankrupt. Have you noticed that your younger doctor just recently moved away to a more rural practice? Or retired early and left medicine altogether? Or that your 50ish doctor also "retired early" and went into another line of work and you now have to establish with another physician?

Is there any wonder we have a problem here? It is perhaps the Internet which has become the biggest offender of all. Since the 1990s, the Internet has evolved into the most powerful medium of informational exchange the world has ever known. It has had far reaching effects upon, and has indeed become the very fabric of Society.

The Good

In a positive light, the Internet has allowed individuals from all over the world to communicate almost instantaneously, sharing their ideas and feelings by Emails and posting boards. We are able to make friends and establish business relationships we would have difficulties making 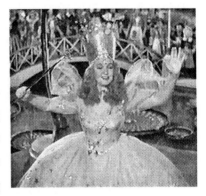 face to face. Previous barriers of socioeconomic status, race, ethnicity, and even language barriers in communication now no longer exist.

The Internet now allows us to shop online, the ability to work from home, and gives each individual an unprecedented freedom of uncensored speech in an anonymous fashion. It has also become perhaps the greatest deflationary business force in the history of mankind. Goods, services, and information are now are bought and sold instantaneously and globally, with the winner usually being the lucky consumer getting if not the best price, at least a very competitive one.

The Net has also now profoundly changed our societal balance of power. Celebrities are now far less powerful, and political figures are under more scrutiny than ever. These individuals now have much less power than they do in real life. Web searches like Google bring up more information regarding any subject than anyone would ever care to read, much less learn or assimilate.

Geeks, nerds, and hackers have become much more powerful with their knowledge of the mechanics of the Internet. Many of the enclaves of power in our world are now easily and anonymously ridiculed, as the geeks are now on a more equal footing than their enemies. Opinions can be expressed without fear of ridicule and allows others with similar points of view a validation. Far more damage can be dished out on the net than in a face to face encounter. The mighty Internet pen continues to trump the sword in almost any twenty-first century fistfight.

The Bad

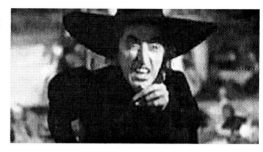

The dark side of the Net seems to lie in somewhat hidden observations. In America, we have another disease now to contend with-along with substance addiction---that of the "cyberjunkie". This is the overweight individual who spends far too much time on his or her computer than is needed to enhance his lifestyle. Time sitting in front of a computer screen could far more profitably be spent in exercise burning caloric activity and has significantly enhanced waistline and derriere expansion. This time away from family and loved ones has insidiously contributed to lack of human interaction, and has subtly allowed our interpersonal relationships to be less well developed than they would be otherwise.

& The Ugly

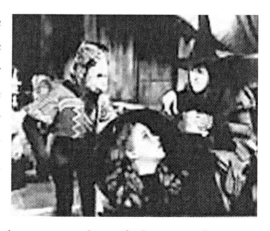

An even darker side of the Net lies in the ease by which illegal or socially unacceptable ideas can be so easily and pervasively disseminated to every user on the Internet. Child pornography, neo-Naziism, and medical quackery have no fear of censorship. Lies, deception, and ripoff schemes are legion. It has become much more difficult for us to differentiate between truth, opinion, fantasy, and even criminal deception. Not only is the average consumer bombarded on a daily basis with filth, sometimes it seems it is almost impossible to escape from their reaches.

Today, all of us as medical consumers are very hungry for information. We peruse the Net in hopes of learning as much as we can, and often do learn a great deal. However, whether or not what we learn is verifiable truth or misleading fiction is often based on the author's intent to sell you a product or service. Lack of censorship is what is missing, because we have a constitutional right to free speech. We have a tendency to believe or want to believe what is in print on the Web. After all, it has to be true, or they wouldn't allow it there, right? The sad truth is there are no Internet police, and medical scams are rampant. It seems any product will help us loose weight, make our skin more beautiful, enhance our sexuality, cure cancer, or ameliorate hot flashes. There seems to always be something out there which is miraculous, and *we want to believe it.*

The Internet Generated Office Visit

I recall an office visit many years ago from one of my highly intelligent, net savvy patients who had not had a menstrual period in over a decade asking me if I would order for her a special "saliva" test to see if she was menopausal. She was in her late forties, and was feeling miserable with hot flashes and night sweats, using "natural" products. She demanded I send her saliva to an Idaho commune where it could be analyzed to determine her "hormone status", just like all the magazines tell perimenopausal women to do. After a full discussion of this request and other (blood) testing available, she still insisted I do this. Three weeks later the results arrived in my office. Yes, the tests all concluded, *she was post-menopausal.* The cost to her from the Idaho lab.: $575, none of which her insurance paid for! In my opinion, this was a preposterous and inappropriate means of evaluating a patient's endocrine status. How did she discover this "revolutionary" new test was available? You guessed it......the Internet.

In America, we now have the best educated in addition to affluent population in our nation's history. Whether or not we are the healthiest generation is somewhat debatable. There is no question we are living longer. Advances in medicine with respect to vaccinations, infectious disease, sanitation, pharmacology, and childbirth safety have all contributed to this remarkable achievement in human longevity.

In 1850, the average life expectancy of a woman in America was age 49, so most women never even lived to reach the age of menopause, which averages age 51 or so. (Menopause is the age at which a woman first experiences a loss of menstrual periods for 12 consecutive months.) Therefore, menopausal medicine is a relatively new specialty among medical disciplines and has evolved by necessity of quality of life for millions of women.

The 2000s Perfect Menopausal Storm: We Don't Mean Hurricanes Either!

Baby boomers are the American generation born between 1946-1964. Many of these women are now reaching menopause, exactly when the Internet is blossoming into a communication medium which has never been 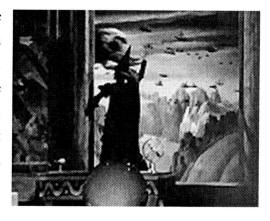 in existence before. The problem lies is that many of them are so hungry for information about the menopause, any information at all, they will devour anything written about this subject they can find without checking its origin. The average layperson Southeby's auction participant would have great difficulty discriminating between a genuine Rembrandt painting and a counterfeit one. The same is true on the Internet regarding complex medical issues.

The advertising media byword now is "natural". It seems that anytime a vendor of Product X can somehow claim their product is "natural", it signifies superiority over conventional prescription pharmaceuticals in effectiveness and safety, when nothing is further from the truth. Alcohol, nicotine, arsenic, mercury, carbon monoxide, and lead are all natural in our environment, but none of them are safe! Just because a medication or supplement is labeled "natural" does NOT mean it is safer than a product created in a laboratory.

Bio-Identical Hormones - Having It Your Way- (It Doesn't Mean Filling Your Prescriptions at Burger King)

The term "*bio-identical hormones*", also known as "natural hormones", has become popular in recent years. This term has been utilized by scientists and health-care providers to signify hormones which are chemically identical duplicates to those produced in the ovaries and other organs. These hormones are available in well tested, FDA approved prescription brand medications, and can be supplied in patches, pills, creams, and gels. Consult your healthcare professional. After all you are not visiting a drive-through restaurant and ordering a cheeseburger.

Unfortunately, the public has come to believe instead that the term bio-identical hormones refers to custom compounded recipes containing one or more of various hormones in different amounts, which are not commercially available, and have to be individually mixed by the pharmacist.

The problem lies in the fact that preparation methods vary from one pharmacist and other, and from one pharmacy to another, making patients receive inconsistent amounts of medication. Also, there are significant safety issues with varying inactive ingredients, reliable sterility, batch to batch differences, and freedom from contaminants.

As such, these products can present a significant risk to the consumer. There is no scientific evidence or documentation these medications are absorbed appropriately or they achieve predictable blood levels for the desired biologic response. Also, your drug benefit plan may or may not pay for a medication not on its formulary. Even if it does, this does not mean it is medically appropriate. In other words, just because the triple decker cheeseburger or chocolate milk shake tasted good doesn't mean it's good for you!

In point of fact, there is virtually almost always more evidence that a pharmacologic preparation is safer than an over-the-counter product. This is because pharmaceutical manufacturers must submit their product to strict testing over thousands of patient over a period of usually years in order to obtain FDA (Food and Drug Administration) approval. Safety and efficacy data are a matter of record and are available in the package insert. FDA monitoring insures purity, and distribution is closely tracked to prevent counterfeiting of the product. Adverse effects of these products are submitted to the FDA itself who regulates these medications.

Do manufacturers of supplements and compounded hormones have to follow any of these requirements? No! Do these alternative products work and are they really safe? Maybe so and maybe not on both issues. We need to see their data, which usually does not exist in a quality of credible scientific documentation to pass accepted FDA approval of the product itself.

Do I believe in Complimentary, Alternative, and Homeopathic (CAHM) Medical Therapy? Yes, absolutely, but it won't be as good as the real thing. If I didn't, I wouldn't have written Chapter 9 in this book on CAHM. More and more credible research is being published about CAHM.

Can't They Just Test My Hormone Levels and Find Out What I Need? (AKA We're Off To See The Wizard…….. the Wonderful Wizard of Saliva?)

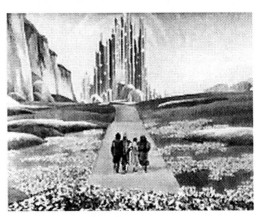

Saliva testing has proven neither accurate nor reliable in the determination of the "right amount" of hormone or combination of hormones necessary for a woman, if they are necessary at all. Prominent women's magazines always seem to advocate the menopausal or perimenopausal female patient should all have hormonal levels checked in her blood. Unfortunately, blood levels of hormones have the drawback of varying tremendously dependent upon the time the day they are drawn. Unlike other hormone levels in medicine, desired hormonal levels in postmenopausal patients have not yet been established. *More importantly, any individual woman's comfort level may not be related at all with her absolute hormonal measurements.* That is not to say that there is not some intrinsic value in blood testing of specific patients under certain clinical circumstances.

For these reasons, the North American Menopause Society has stated in written opinion that it *does not* recommend any bio-identical or custom compounded products over well tested prescription medication for the vast majority women. It also *does not* recommend saliva testing to determine hormone levels either.

Straight Talk

Women desire and should seek out straight talk from their health care practitioners, whom should be consulted regularly in performance of routine screening tests….. such as mammography, breast exams, pelvic exams, Pap smears, bone densities, colonoscopies, and blood screening tests. Those practitioners should in turn be well versed in each patient's historical, physical, and laboratory findings. These findings should help provide a unique patient profile of disease risk factors as you pass from midlife into your menopausal years. You should be able to ask intelligent questions and obtain real answers about various treatments and their alternatives. It is strongly recommended that you allow your healthcare professional to perform preventative and diagnostic testing that is usual and customary for your specific age group and medical conditions. Your quality of life and indeed your longevity itself depend on it.

It is well known that women die everyday from the medical condition associated with the menopause known as estrogen deficiency, which manifests itself in the form of osteoporosis, decreased cognitive function, depression, decreased immunity, and a host of other conditions. The decision of whether or not hormonal replacement (HT) is the right choice for a specific woman is a complex one, and for each patient the answer may be slightly different. Ultimately, it is the patient herself who should make an informed choice to take or not to take it, depending on each one's individual health histories and need for quality of life.

It has been said that in America only about 15% of patients who should take HT for longevity and life quality are really taking it, through either lack of objective information or professional care. Not everyone, of course, should be taking it. Patients who decide to go the route of taking HT do live on average a documented seven to nine years longer and look much younger compared to their peers. They also have a much higher quality of life than those who do not. I sincerely believe that whichever route the patient goes, there are risks, and in fact, there may be more risks associated with *not taking therapy than in taking it.*

The Frustration

I have seen several well meaning but misguided family physicians try to discontinue HT on my patients, not for valid medical reasons, but for no other good reason than what they read in the newspaper headlines, written by laypersons. This is after my or another physician's often exhaustive evaluation of specific health details and risk factors for each patient, relative to their desire for quality of life. Once these patients stop HT, a few of them can tolerate absence of therapy, but a lot of them end back up in my office wondering why they feel so miserable. As a certified NAMS Menopausal Practitioner, it is my opinion that it should rarely be a split second decision either to initiate or terminate HT, provided proper thought has been administered.

However, we are not here to sell anyone a product, be it medication, strategies, or remedies. We have no hidden agenda. This book is chaos free and commercial free, low fat, and totally natural, straight from the authors' hearts. Collectively speaking, we have been there and done menopause, on both sides of the white coat. Our focus is to present straightforward balanced information from the most credible updated sources available, based on valid scientific studies without all the academic lingo, so that it maybe read, understood, and evaluated by women of all educational levels. I do each this each and every day in my private practice of gynecology in South Florida.

You Are Worth It!

It is my belief that the best medicine we can utilize is that which we know to be safe and effective. My attitude is show us the data to substantiate your product claims. After all, why should we put more investigation in the purchase of a toaster than into a medication we ingest for months, perhaps years? After all, aren't we worth it?

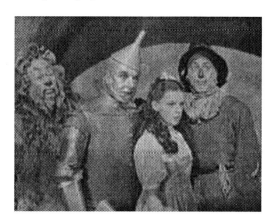

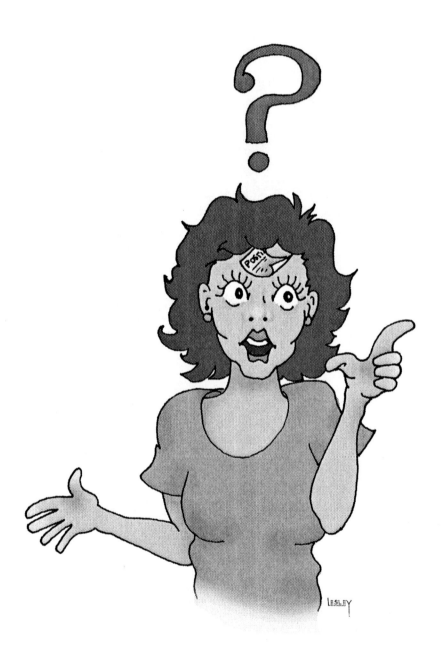

You can't remember where the post it note is,
and what you put on it!

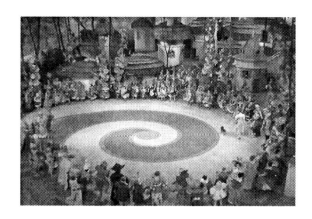

Chapter 2:

The Menopause and the End of Reproductive Function: A New Beginning

By Neil C. Boland, M.D., F.A.C.O.G.

The Big Picture

The female reproductive system begins to age at birth with a set finite number of eggs known as oocytes. Then, at the age of first menstruation (also known as menarche) which occurs usually between age 10 and 16, a woman begins to ovulate approximately every month or so. An egg is lost if fertilization is not achieved with pregnancy. These oocytes, present in the ovaries, gradually decline in number over the next 50 years or so.

This aging of the female reproductive system begins at birth, and proceeds at different rates in different women. Therefore, simply a woman's chronologic age is a poor indicator of the beginning or end of her transition into menopause.

For many years, the subject of menopause has been quite a taboo subject, being relegated to either silent anxiety or quiet whispers between friends. It was even associated with psychiatric illness, as well as decreased sexual desire, deep depression, and severe mood swings. Fortunately, however, many of these negative stereotypes have begun to fall by the wayside, largely due to widespread media attention and popular books and magazines. Today menopause is now seen as a natural part of the aging process with both positive and negative aspects. Women have now begun to discuss menopause and and its clinical aspects quite openly with one another as well as their healthcare practitioners.

Why is the subject of menopause so relevant in today's world? Menopause is an extremely important public health issue, predominantly because of three factors: 1) it will eventually affect every woman, 2) more postmenopausal women are alive than ever before in the history the world, and 3) longevity in the United States is at an all-time high. Today in America, a woman who reaches age 54 can expect to reach age 84.3. The average female life expectancy is 79.7 years. Approximately two thirds of the total U.S. population is expected to live to age 85 or longer. In fact, most women will now live at least a full third of their life as a postmenopausal patient.

Important Menopausal Definitions

The term *premenopause* refers to that time in a woman's life, which precedes menopause. This term has become so confusing that it has been recommended this name be abandoned.

Patients frequently and inaccurately confuse the term menopause as an event that occurs over 20 years or so, when in actuality, the term menopause refers to a specific point in time. *Spontaneous (or natural) menopause* is defined as 12 consecutive months without any menstrual bleeding whatsoever. Spontaneous menopause occurs naturally somewhere between 40-58, with an average age of 51.4 years, with a median age of onset of menopausal transition of 47.5 years, which is called the *climacteric* (see below).

Induced menopause is the absence of menstrual function brought about by either surgical removal of the ovaries, chemotherapy, or pelvic radiation for treatment of malignancy. For example, if the patient has had a total abdominal hysterectomy with removal of both ovaries, then she is said to have undergone a surgically induced menopause. If her body is accustomed to being in an environment in which estrogen is available, she will experience estrogen deficiency symptoms almost immediately, unless some type of hormonal replacement occurs. It is very important to mention at this point that any vaginal bleeding which occurs after these 12 months have elapsed from her last menstruation should be reported to her gynecologist for evaluation to rule out genital tract cancer.

Climacteric era, also known as the *perimenopausal era, refers to the time in transition that a woman spends between her reproductive and her nonreproductive state (of menopause). This is a time elapsed process and not a specific moment in time. This climacteric period lasts approximately 4 years. It is during this time that specific hormonal changes occur which are mainly a gradual decrease in serum (blood) estrogen levels, which is manufactured by the ovary, and an increase in serum follicle stimulating hormone levels (FSH), which is manufactured by the pituitary gland deep in the brain. It is important to note, however, that what is commonly thought of as menopausal symptoms usually, but not always, begin slowly in the climacteric era.*

These menopausal-like symptoms include, but are not limited to: hot flashes, night sweats, skin dryness, mood swings, depression, insomnia, memory changes, inability to concentrate, vaginal dryness, decreased sexual drive, fatigue, and changes in menstrual timing and flow amount. The duration and severity of the symptoms seems to vary from woman to woman. In some women, these symptoms can last for no more than several months, and others find the symptoms can last for years, if not decades.

Changes in menstrual bleeding patterns during the climacteric era can include either heavier or lighter flow, a lengthening of the time between periods, or skipped periods altogether. Most women do notice some change in menstrual pattern; however, only 10% of them or less stop menstruation abruptly without menstrual regularity prior to menopause.

The term postmenopausal applies to any time which is after 12 months have elapsed from the last menses, or any time immediately after surgical removal of the ovaries.

The term *premature menopause* can be defined as any menopause which occurs prior to the age of 40, whether it be spontaneous or induced. If this condition occurs, it should be reported to your health care practitioner, and a diligent search should be made to determine if other endocrine problems coexist, such as an underactive thyroid gland (hypothyroidism). When one endocrine organ is under active, it is more likely that others will be as well.

The term *premature ovarian failure* is used to describe insufficient enough ovarian function under age 40 that the woman no longer has periods. This can result from temporary causes such as high stress levels, eating disorders, or over exercising. Permanent causes may result from either genetic abnormalities or from autoimmune diseases.

The term *temporary menopause* is mentioned only because it has been recommended to be abandoned by the North American Menopause Society.

Normal Hormonal Changes Around Menopause

In late midlife, as ovulation becomes more irregular, the cyclical changes in estrogen and progesterone present in a normal menstrual cycle become disrupted. As a result, women experience irregular vaginal bleeding, episodes of skipping periods altogether, and eventually no periods at all. During this transitionary phase (or climacteric), painful sexual intercourse may arise associated with lack of estrogen in the vagina and vulva.

During the reproductive years, the ovary is the body's major source of estrogen. During the climacteric years, a marked reduction in ovarian estrogen secretion occurs. Therefore, many menopausal-like symptoms (as outlined above) occur during this climacteric time. The greatest fall in estrogen occurs in the first year subsequent to absence of menses for 12 months. A more gradual decline follows just after the menopause. A common blood test utilized to determine if a woman is in ovarian failure or menopause is that of follicle stimulating hormone, also known as FSH level.

FSH is produced by the pituitary gland deep in the brain. If this hormonal level exceeds 10 ng per ml., it is said that the patient is in ovarian failure, and if over 30, is post-menopausal. FSH is a fascinating hormone because its elevation is one of the very first signs of the impending climacteric era. Women report waking up with hot flashes at 3 A.M. somewhere between ages 35-45, and this is indicative of a drop in estrogen, which accompanies the rise in serum FSH.

A second hormone called progesterone, normally present in higher levels in the second half of a reproductive woman's menstrual cycle, is also present in normal levels during the climacteric time. The levels drop, however, as a woman approaches menopause.

A third hormone, testosterone, is also manufactured by the ovary adrenal gland, and fat cell conversion during the reproductive years. This is exactly the same hormone that is manufactured in the testicles. It has been discovered that the normal cyclical peak in testosterone, commonly found elevated around ovulation in younger women, is absent in older regularly cycling women between ages 43-47. Conflicting data suggest that there may be transient drops in testosterone around the time of menopause, to be followed by normalization of testosterone levels in patients after menopause. The postmenopausal ovary then continues to produce testosterone and another androgen-like hormone called androstenedione. Total testosterone, but not bioavailable (free) testosterone, levels actually appear to increase with age, stabilizing to premenopausal levels by age 70.

It is noted that surgical menopause (removal of the ovaries) immediately results in lower testosterone levels. Both free and total testosterone levels remain at 40-50% lower levels than in women who have not undergone surgical menopause.

Factors Affecting The Age of Menopause

In general, while the age of first menstruation (menarche) has become younger and younger over the last several centuries, the age of menopause has remained relatively unchanged. This is despite improving worldwide nutrition and reduction of infectious disease. No established link has been discovered between the age of menopause and the use or avoidance of birth control pills, age of onset of first menses, socioeconomic, or marital status.

However, data does exist for the association of age of onset of menopause at both earlier and later times than average (51.4 years).

Earlier Menopause Than Average:

1)   History of never having been pregnant

2)   Epilepsy (especially with high lifetime seizure frequency)

3)   Previous treatment of childhood cancer by radiation of the pelvis and or certain types of chemotherapy (alkylating agents)

4) Smoking, which tends to shift menopause earlier, approximately by 1 1/2 -2 years, as nicotine itself is an anti-estrogen chemical substance. This does appear to be dose related, as to number of cigarettes smoked, multiplied by years of smoking.

Later Menopause Than Average:

1) Having more than one pregnancy

2) High cognitive scores in childhood in education

3) Obesity (higher body mass index scores).

The Numbers Tell The Story

In the year 2000, it was estimated that almost 46 million United States women were postmenopausal. Of this number, about 40 million of them were older than age 51. It is estimated that by the year 2020, there will be more than 50 million American women, who are postmenopausal, and virtually all the baby boomer generation will be joining the club. Worldwide, by the year 2025, the number of postmenopausal women will be expected to exceed 1.1 billion, as life expectancy will rise from 72 to 82 years in more developed countries.

The economic power of this demographic menopausal group of patients will be immense and unprecedented long before year 2020. The ramifications for elderly worldwide healthcare will be extremely significant in almost all countries throughout the world. Since eventually all women will likely face menopause and the changes that it will impose on their health, it is imperative that each woman become as knowledgeable as possible about this subject. Her longevity and quality-of-life will very likely depend upon the knowledge she possesses, as well as the relationship she has established with her individual healthcare provider community.

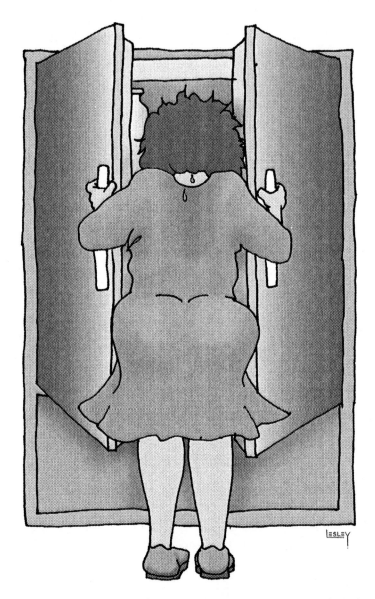

You buy a large double door fridge to put your head in!

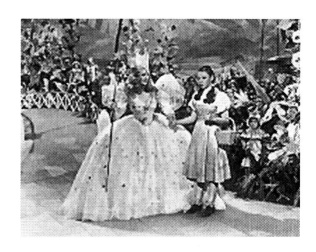

Chapter 3:

The Effects of Menopause On Your Health: What You Need To Know Now

By Neil C. Boland, M.D. , F.A.C.O.G.

The Times They Are A Changing

As a woman progresses through perimenopausal transition into menopause, an obvious change is that of menstrual irregularity and beyond this, a total absence of periods. As outlined before, the median age for menses to stop completely is around 51. Beginning around an average age of 47, a woman may notice lighter or heavier bleeding, perhaps more prolonged bleeding, skipped periods, or even no changes in menses at all. OB-GYN specialists label this specific type of menstrual pattern as *dysfunctional uterine bleeding*, also known as DUB, provided that the bleeding itself is not the result of tumor growth, infection, or pregnancy.

It is important to note that a significant decline in fertility occurs in women progressively after age 30, and continues to decline on into menopause. Although her fertility is significantly decreased, a woman may still become pregnant even during the perimenopausal or climacteric era. Therefore, contraception is still important for women in this age group, unless she has had a previous hysterectomy, tubal ligation, or presently has a partner with a vasectomy.

Is it safe to use birth control pills between ages 40-55? Absolutely, provided the patient is a non-smoker, and is otherwise healthy, with no history of hypertension, elevated blood cholesterol values, heart attack, diabetes, hepatitis, estrogen dependent malignancy, history of thrombophlebitis (extremity blood clot), or pulmonary embolus (blood clot in the lungs). In fact, some of the healthiest and happiest patients I have my practice take birth control pills in this age category for contraception, relief of hot flashes, and bleeding control. However, this should always be done under the supervision of your healthcare provider and at his or her discretion.

Postmenopausal Bleeding (Bleeding After The Change)

In order to rule out malignancy, it is always very important for you to report to your physician any vaginal bleeding noted once menopause has occurred. Most postmenopausal bleeding can represent a host of benign origins:

1) Uterine fibroids (benign muscle tumors)

2) Endometrial polyps (benign uterine lining growths)

3) Cervical polyps

4) Endometrial hyperplasia (benign build up of the uterine lining)

5) Atrophic vaginitis (thin, dry, and easily traumatized vagina)

6) A normal uterine lining adjustment to hormonal replacement therapy

7) Possibly expected and normal withdrawal bleeding from certain hormonal replacement therapy regimens

Approximately 70% of women who initiate certain types of hormonal replacement therapy (HT), will experience the temporary inconvenience of intermittent vaginal bleeding. This is to be anticipated as normal, and is not meant to be heavy or prolonged and should disappear in several months. Specific types of HT are more likely to cause bleeding than others, and you should consult your physician about this. However, once you are adjusted with your medication, no further bleeding should occur.

Unfortunately, other origins of postmenopausal bleeding can be also either premalignant or malignant, such as endometrial carcinoma (cancer), atypical endometrial hyperplasia (precancer of the uterine lining) , primary carcinoma of the fallopian tube, or cervical carcinoma. Tell your doctor about the bleeding. The workup of evaluation will likely include a transvaginal ultrasound to determine the uterine lining thickness, a Pap smear if it has not been recently performed, and an endometrial lining sampling procedure (also called an endometrial biopsy).

Most patients are quite surprised to learn that these endometrial origins of cancer are approximately 50% *reduced* below taking no medication at all in patients taking HT correctly. *The catch here is government approved (FDA approved) HT.* If you're taking medication from a compounding pharmacy, you might be shocked to learn that there is no data available that you are not increasing your risk of uterine cancer. In patients using government approved oral or transdermal (skin applied) HT formulations, the incidence of endometrial hyperplasia is less than 1%.

When you receive any medication at your pharmacy, you will get with it something written called the *package insert*, which is both a blessing and a curse. While it gives the reader an incredible amount of data about the medication and its side effects, it can also present outdated information. For example, most estrogen products have a warning about the increased incidence of endometrial cancer if used, which is true is a patient is taking unopposed estrogen without progesterone in a patient with an intact uterus. The problem is that this warning is still listed inappropriately even on inserts for *combination* estrogen/ progesterone meds. As such, the poor patient is scared out of her wits either due to reading such misinformation, or about a side effect which occurs a very tiny percentage of the time. The patient throws her medication away or doesn't take it, and then goes back to the internet looking for something "natural", only to be ripped off again, all very discouraging, to say the least!

Is It Hot In Here Or What? Vasomotor Symptoms

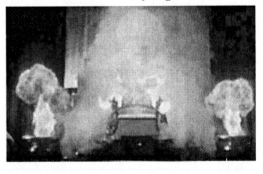

One on the hallmarks of perimenopause and menopause itself is that of the hot flash. These are also known as hot flushes, or vasomotor symptoms. Night sweats are simply hot flashes that occur with sweat during sleep. I want you to take heart in the statistic that approximately 25% of women in the United States report feeling no perimenopausal symptoms whatsoever. However, for those women who do experience the symptoms, it can be simply just an annoyance to a severe impediment to their quality-of-life.

The culprit in the generation of hot flashes is a sudden drop in estrogen levels. The estrogen drop itself sends a message to your brain (the hypothalamus) that something is wrong. In turn, your brain releases, a hormone called norepinephrine, also known as adrenaline, which triggers the so-called "fight or flight" syndrome. This goes back to when we were cave women or men being attacked by a wild animal, and this gets our heart racing, and blood pressure elevated. We sometimes experience a rapid heartbeat as "flutters" also known as palpitations. Increases in heart rate of 7 to 15 beats per minute can be noted, and remain elevated for at least three minutes. In turn, this causes arteries in your upper body, such as head or neck, to expand or dilate and all of a sudden, we feel as if the room is 110° Fahrenheit. YIKES! Sometimes, the flashes are even followed by chills. The temperature itself can rise as much as one to seven degrees Centigrade in the fingers and toes where it is the most pronounced. In general, hot flashes last anywhere from one to five minutes.

This seems to be a consistent pattern of hot flashes within the same woman's metabolic system. These flashes can occur as frequently as every hour or as infrequently as every week or month. In many women they appear to occur with repetitive patterns, peaking in the early evening hours. The severity of hot flashes, is usually simply mild or moderate. However, at least 10% of women notice severe enough hot flashes to be completely debilitated by them.

Ethnic differences have also been described among different racial groups of women in the severity of hot flash prevalence. Early data from the Study of Women's Health Across the Nation (SWAN) Study in the United States reveal that African-American women report the highest frequency of hot flashes at (45.6%.) This is followed by Hispanic women (35.4%), Caucasian women (31.2%), Chinese Americans (20.5%), and Japanese-American (17.6%).

More recent studies have tended to suggest that a higher body mass index (BMIs greater than 27 kg./ square meter) may actually be a better positive predictor of hot flashes than her ethnic origin. Older theories suggested that the more obese a woman was, the higher her estrogen level, due to her extra fat cells manufacturing excess estrogen from hormonal precursors. However, the effect of extra estrogen in these fatter women seems to be outweighed by her extra fat insulation, making her have a higher core temperature, and thus more hot flashes.

Night sweats frequently wake us, and they make it quite difficult to get back to sleep. This leaves us bleary-eyed and sleep deprived in the morning, further contributing to lack of mental agility and a distinct inability to concentrate and focus on our daily tasks. It seems astounding to me how many patients report this mental fog, or decline in mental functioning, which will be covered in a Chapter 8.

Decline in estrogen levels also contributes to a decline in serotonin, which is the brain's own so-called 'feel-good' hormone. Conversely, rises in estrogen, contribute to rises in serotonin. Serotonin is that magic hormone, or neurotransmitter, which is elevated, when we eat chocolate or take medication such as Prozac or Zoloft. It is this drop in estrogen levels, which triggers the drop in serotonin, and all of a sudden, we become irritable, anxious, depressed, and are unable to remember where we put our car keys.

In addition to serotonin levels diminishing, other brain neurochemicals drop as well. Endorphins are our body's natural mood regulators and painkillers and they drop as well. It is these endomorphins which are released our body by heavy physical activity, creating the so-called "runner's high".

These hot flashes, or vasomotor symptoms, occur most commonly in the first two years after the last period, and then decline slowly over time. The duration of hot flashes can occur anywhere from an average of six months to two years. *It is not widely known that flashes can continue for five, ten, twenty years or longer in many patients, and they can continue to contribute to decline in quality-of-life for many women.* Available prescription treatment and CAHM (complimentary, alternative, and homeopathic medication) do not actually cure hot flashes per se, but they simply make the flashes tolerable. Eventually, all flashes will stop spontaneously. However, there remains no reliable method of determination when exactly this will occur in any particular woman.

Other Origins of Hot Flashes

Estrogen deficiency is only one of many causes of the hot flash. Other origins include pancreatic tumors, autoimmune disorders, many infections, epilepsy, thyroid disease, leukemia, and also very rare tumors such as carcinoid syndrome and phaeochromocytoma. Hot flashes can also be common side effects of drugs such as tamoxifen (Novadex) and raloxifene (Evista).

What factors could also be triggering hot flashes, other than reasons mentioned above?

1) Cigarette smoking actually lowers your estrogen level by inactivating a lot of it and can trigger hot flashes. One study demonstrated that the higher number of cigarettes smoked daily, the higher the number of hot flashes.

2) It is also been shown that the more sedentary a woman is and the less her physical activity level, the more likely it is she will experience hot flashes. Conversely, the more a woman exercises, the less likely she will have hot flashes.

3) Higher ambient (air) temperatures seem also to be correlated with higher hot flash incidence, and lower air temperatures with less. In other words, if it is hot in the room, you may notice more hot flashes. (So ladies, let's drop the thermostat when he's not looking!).

4) Certain foods and beverages, such as those foods containing MSG (monosodium glutamate), caffeine, or alcohol have only anecdotally been shown to trigger hot flashes, but not clinically proven.

Sleeping Difficulties

It is extremely important that all of us get enough sleep. The amount of sleep each of us needs varies with the individual, dependent upon how much will maintain mental alertness for us during waking hours. It has been estimated at least one third to one half of menopausal or menopausal women have impaired sleeping. These menopausal patients are twice as likely to use sleeping aids is the general population. Not enough sleep or poor quality sleep contributes to mood changes, inability to concentrate, and even irritability. The origin of the sleeping difficulties can be multiple: vasomotor symptoms, depression, sleep apnea, drug and alcohol use and abuse, caffeine in liquid intake, bladder irritability, arthritis, fibromyalgia, a host of neurological, cardiac, and gastrointestinal diseases. Then there is of course stress, which unfortunately is much more common in women at this point in their lives due to stress, divorce, or family care giving issues.

Urinary Tract Infections and Incontinence

Studies show that as women age, they are more likely to become incontinent, but this is not contingent upon the onset of menopause per se. Approximately 10-30% of all American women are incontinent. One origin of this incontinence can be related to previous childbearing injuries resulting in stretching of the pelvic floor and abnormal bladder positioning, resulting in abnormal pressure formation on the bladder and urethra. This is called *stress urinary incontinence,* and is actually the most common in women during perimenopause.

A second form of urinary incontinence, called *urge incontinence*, is due to increasing irritability of the bladder wall, and is very frequent in postmenopausal patients. This results in spontaneous bladder emptying with a full bladder, and almost always causes nocturia, or frequent trips to the bathroom interrupting sleep, which is exactly what the older patient does not need.

Frequently, stress and urge incontinence coexist, and create a third variety, called *mixed urinary incontinence.* A common misconception among patients is that all they need is a "bladder tack" operation, and this should take care of the problem. Multiple types of surgical procedures can improve significantly or even eliminate stress incontinence, as well as pelvic floor tightening exercises, called Kegal's exercises. However, improvement in urge incontinence is generally with medication and bladder retraining, not surgery. Severe mixed incontinences frequently require both surgical and medical therapy.

We will not go into a fourth variety of incontinence having to do with damage to the sphincter muscle between the bladder and the urethra, called *intrinsic sphincter deficiency*, or ISD. Other causes of urinary incontinence can be recurrent bladder infections, diuretics, some tranquilizers, obesity, and other medical conditions such as Parkinson's disease, multiple sclerosis, stroke, and diabetes.

It is important to point out that *any* incontinence or urinary complaint is abnormal, and not necessarily the result of the aging process. This should be pointed out to your healthcare provider. Unfortunately, all too often, the menopausal patient is too embarrassed to discuss this problem with anyone and resorts instead to the chronic use of absorbency napkins, pads, or diapers. These wet diaper-like materials confer a wick like wetness to the vulva, and trap bacteria which can in turn, enter the urethra more easily, causing bladder infections, also known as cystitis. Bladder infections and vaginitis are much more common in the menopausal patient, due to a higher pH (due to dropping estrogen levels) of the vagina, urethra, and bladder. Unfortunately as well, incontinent patients often decrease their fluid intake, which makes the problem even worse.

The incidence of stress urinary incontinence has been hypothesized to be worsened due to estrogen deficiency. However, a recent study, has shown that estrogen therapy itself or HT actually makes stress incontinence slightly worse, which is contrary to what we would expect.

The incidence of fecal (rectal) incontinence been shown to be present in approximately 15-20% of women with urinary incontinence. This incontinence of stool or gas is also more likely to be present in a patient with neuromuscular dysfunction from childbearing or other neurological origins. It has also been hypothesized that since the anorectal area contains an abundance of estrogen receptors, that estrogen deficiency may contribute to fecal incontinence in the post-menopausal patient.

Vulvovaginal Complaints

As discussed above, the drop in estrogen associated with menopause frequently causes a chronic vulvar and vaginal dryness called vulvovaginal atrophy or atrophic vaginitis. This causes chronic labial itching, and more frequent episodes of a malodorous discharge called bacterial vaginosis, also called BV. Frequently, alleviation of these symptoms is possible with simply topical estrogen creams or pills. Bacterial vaginosis is treated with various types of antibiotics.

Probably the most common menopausal complaint besides yeast infections in presentation to the gynecologist's office is that of increasingly severe painful intercourse, which is due to a thinning of the diameter of the vaginal walls with shrinkage of the entire vaginal capacity. This is to say that the pre-menopausal estrogenized vagina is thicker, more elastic, with more ridges or rugae than the vagina of the postmenopausal patient. The atrophic vagina is much more prone to trauma, and even bleeding with intercourse. Fortunately, this is quite well responsive to estrogen therapy. Atrophic vaginitis symptoms are also less common in the patient who is frequently sexually active, because intercourse promotes increased blood supply to the pelvis.

Vulvar yeast infections, also called candida infections, are also common in the postmenopausal patient, primarily due to moisture from incontinence, sweating, use of non-cotton underwear or antibiotics, steroids, or immunosuppressive medication. Also, since the incidence of obesity is dramatically increasing in America, so is the incidence of diabetes, which not only increases neuromuscular dysfunction, and urination, but also seems to suppress the immune system. It is imperative that the healthcare professional address the root cause of the candida infection, as well as the yeast itself, or almost certainly the patient will return with the same complaint.

Changes In The Central Nervous System

Multiple CNS alterations can and do occur frequently in the perimenopausal or postmenopausal patient. These changes can include headaches, mood swings, changes in cognitive function, and depression.

As women go through the hormonal fluctuations associated with falling estrogen levels as they age, they frequently incur very worrisome symptoms, such as fatigue, irritability, tearfulness, insomnia, and impaired memory and concentration. Sleep deprivation in and of itself can be a significant contributory factor.

Is important to make a distinction between PMS (also called premenstrual tension syndrome, luteal phase dysphoria, or premenstrual dysphoric disorder) and the menopause. PMS can appear at any age a woman is capable of menstruation, and has been discovered, and indeed validated as a legitimate medical diagnosis in recent years, thought to be a deficiency of the hormone serotonin in the brain and spinal

35

cord during the latter half of the menstrual cycle. There seems to be an increase in PMS-like symptoms in some women at the onset of the perimenopause. Menopausal patients do not incur significant hormonal fluctuations and do not get PMS.

Also, during the perimenopause, the severity and incidence of menstrual migraine headaches seem to increase due to hormonal fluctuations. Migraine headaches occur in approximately 18% of menstrating female population. Once menopause is occurred, and menses have stopped for 12 consecutive months, the incidence of migraines drops to that of the male population.

Mood disturbances in the menopausal patient can be due to a host of origins such as nutritional deficiencies, stress, other age-related chronic illnesses or medications prescribed them, recurrence or new onset depression, hypothyroidism, or changes in socioeconomic status.

Although many women do report the menopause affords them a period of fulfillment and happiness compared with other times in their lives, aging can become stressful and difficult. Changes in body image and self-esteem cause many women to reflect upon the meaning and purpose of their lives, along with their own mortality.

Depression, along with anxiety, occurs at a much higher rate among women than men. It is also true that depressive episodes can recur during the perimenopause. However, the vast majority of women undergo menopausal transition without significant psychiatric problems. A review of the literature reveals there is *no* substantial evidence that menopause per se puts women at increased risk for depression, which is good news.

Cognition is a complex neurological interaction between various areas of the brain are involved with short and long-term memory, concentration, information processing, and recall. Estrogen, progesterone, and testosterone hormones all participate in modulating aspects of brain function.   Multiple areas the brain have hormone receptors for all three hormones.   Estrogen deficiency seems to increase the activity of a brain enzyme called *monoamine oxidase*, which seems to facilitate or enhance the breakdown of neurotransmitters which is detrimental. These neurotransmitters, such as dopamine, norepinephrine, serotonin, and acetylcholine facilitate cognitive functions involved with memory reasoning and recall.

Previous studies administered to recently menopausal patients have shown as much as a 30% decline in cognitive function, which is objectively measurable.   It is also been shown that the vast majority of this decline improves when hormones are reinitiated.   It is the acutely menopausal patient, such as that with an untreated postsurgery patient with her ovaries removed, that shows the most acute fluctuation in memory, learning, and mood changes.   For further information on cognitive function, please see Chapter 8.

Ocular (Eye) Changes

We are all aware that our visual acuity seems to change as we get older in both men and women. This may be due to alteration of corneal curvature or edema formation, associated with the eyelid or the conjunctiva. As such, contact lens usage may be much more difficult. Many perimenopausal patients resort to reading glasses, due to these visual changes.

Dry eyes are a common complaint in the postmenopausal patient, causing burning, light intolerance, pressure, redness, and scratchiness. It is been postulated as well that dry eye syndrome is directly related to a drop in testosterone levels that occurs with aging. It seems that testosterone exerts an ocular anti-inflammatory effect on the eye.

Estrogen also affords the user in a decrease in cataract formation in the postmenopausal woman. It is known that the incidence of cataracts increase in both men and women as they age.

Dental changes

Low bone mineral density of the bones can be associated with osteoporosis, as we will demonstrate in a subsequent chapter. Unfortunately, this low bone mineral density is also associated with loss of teeth in both upper and lower jaw with need for dentures, and a much higher incidence of periodontal disease. It has been demonstrated that for each 1% per year decrease in body bone mineral density (BMD), there is a *fourfold increase in tooth loss*. In patients using estrogen, progesterone (or a combination of the two) in long term studies, there appears to be a significant reduction of risk of tooth loss. This would imply that prevention and/ or treatment of osteoporosis in the menopausal patient is important in good dental health.

Lack of estrogen associated with menopause can also affect growth and proliferation of the gingival (gum) membrane, thereby increasing gum recession. This, and turn, leads to increased tooth sensitivity and burning in the oral cavity.

Weight Gain

There is _no_ scientific evidence to support the fact that hormonal therapy (HT) is contributory in any way to weight gain during menopause. Instead weight gain is more related to aging itself and to body fat accumulation throughout an individual's adult life. It is well known that body fat percentage increases we grow older, and lean muscle mass decreases, which is made worse by a more sedentary lifestyle.

In the late 1990s, a study was done, called the PEPI Study (Postmenopausal Estrogen/ Progesterone Interventions Trial). This study demonstrated that patients taking estrogen with or without progesterone weighed on average about 2.2 pounds less than a control population after three years of therapy. There was no difference noted in weight between patients taking estrogen only or is taking combination therapy.

Other Effects

Other involved organ systems with the menopause include the cardiovascular system, the skeletal system, the skin, and female sexuality, which will be all be dealt with in subsequent chapters.

Who Should Not Take Hormonal Therapy?

Any patient having any of the following medical conditions contraindicate taking Hormonal Therapy (HT):

(See Chapter 10 for Birth Control Pill Contraindications).

1) Pregnancy

2) Active or History of Deep Venous Thrombosis/ Thrombophlebitis

3) History of Pulmonary Embolus

4) Recent Heart Attack

5) Severe Angina

6) Known Peripheral Vascular Disease

7) History of Stroke or Cerebrovascular Attack (CVA)

8) Untreated Hypertension

9) Present Anticoagulation Therapy

10) Prolonged Hospitalization

11) Recent Surgery Involving Immobilization

12) Liver Dysfunction

13) Hepatic Adenomas

14) Undiagnosed Vaginal Bleeding

15) Some Types of Migraine Headaches

16) History of Ischemic Colitis

17) Most Advanced Diabetic Conditions

18) Advanced or Familial Dyslipidemias

19) Most Estrogen Dependent Neoplasia (Breast or Endometrial Cancer)

Please note the above list did not include either a family history of breast or endometrial cancer, or smoking.

Available Hormonal Prescription Medications (U.S. only products)

Estrogens Products:

Oral (milligram doses)

1) Conjugated Equine Estrogens (Premarin) 0.3, 0.45, 0.625, 0.9, and 1.25. The 2.5 mg. dose is no longer manufactured due to low demand.

2) Synthetic Conjugated Estrogens: (Cenestin) and (Enjuvia) same as Premarin doses.

3) Esterified Estrogens: (Menest) 0.3, 0.625, 1.25, 2.5 mg.

4) 17 Beta-Estradiol: (Estrace) 0.5, 1.0, and 2.0 mg., along with various generic substitutions.

5) Estropipate (Ortho-Est) 0.75, 1.5 mg.

6) Piperazine Estrone Sulfate (Ogen) 0.75, 1.5, 3.0, 6.0 mg.

7) Ethinyl Estradiol (Estinyl) 0.02 and 0.05 mg.

Transdermal Patches (milligram doses):
Note: All patches are twice weekly skin application except Climara, which is once weekly.

*17-Beta Estradiol Matrix :

Alora 0.025, 0.005, 0.075, 0.1 mg.

Climara 0.025, 0.05, 0.075, 0.1 mg.

Esclim (same, add 0.0375 mg)

Vivelle Dot (same, add 0.0375 mg.)

Various Generics: 0.05 and 0.1 mg

*17-Beta Estradiol Reservoir:

Estraderm 0.025, 0.05, and 0.1 mg.

*Topical Transdermal Gel:

Estrogel 0.75 mg of dose metered pump 1.25 mg daily.

*Topical Emulsion:

Estrasorb 0.05 mg with daily application of 2 packets

Vaginal ET Cream Products:

Estrace Vaginal Cream:

2-4 grams / day for 3 weeks, then 1 gram daily.

Premarin Vaginal Cream:

0.5-2.0 grams per day for 3 weeks on, one week off (optional).

Vaginal ET Ring Therapy Products:

Estring: Indwelling vaginal ring, changed every 90 days. Note: This product achieves a *local vaginal effect only* (not a systemic effect), which is very desireable when systemic estrogen is contraindicated.

Femring: Indwelling vaginal ring, changed every 90 days. Note: This product achieves a *systemic effect, not just a vaginal effect.*

Vagifem: Tablets applied vaginally once daily for 2 weeks, then twice weekly. Note: Systemic effect, same as Femring.

Note: Estrogen can also be administered by injections (rarely used) or by insertion of subcutaneous pellet delivery systems. Consult your provider.

Progestin Products:

Oral: (milligram doses)

Medroxyprogesterone Acetate (MPA, or Provera) 2.5, 5, 10 mg.

Norethindrone (Micronor) 0.35 mg

Norethindrone Acetate (NETA, or Aygestin) 5 mg.

Megestrol Acetate (Megace) 20, 40 mg.

Micronized Progesterone, in peanut oil (Prometrium) 100, 200 mg.

Vaginal Progesterone Gel (Prochieve) 4% 45 mg application.

Levonorgestel IUD (Mirena) 5 year usage (see Chapter 10, Question 8).

*****Please note that most of the above medications can be utilized in a pure estrogen and pure progestin co-administration, either continuously daily, or in a cyclic fashion. Consult your health care provider.

Oral Combined Medications (E+P):

Continuous Regimens:

Prempro (Premarin + Provera) 0.3/1.5 mg, 0.45/1.5 mg., 0.625/ 2.5 mg. , and 0.625/5 mg. daily.

FemHRT: 5 mcg. E + 1 mg P daily.

Activella: 1 mg. E + 0.5 mg P daily.

Cyclic Regimens:

Premphase: Premarin 0.625 mg + Provera 5 mg.

Take P daily X 2 weeks, then E+P daily for 2 weeks.

Oral Intermittent Combined Regimen:

PreFest: 1 mg E+ 0.09 mg P. Take 2 days E, then 1 day P, repeat.

Transdermal (Patches) Continous Combined Medications (E+P):

17 Beta- Estradiol + NETA (Combipatch) 0.05 mg E + 0.14 mg. P twice weekly. Also 0.05 mg E + 0.25 mg available.

17 Beta-Estradiol + Levonorgestrel (Climara Pro) 0.045 mg E + 0.0015 mg. P once weekly.

Please note again that all these medications have to be taken appropriately as prescribed by your provider. If not, the patient may experience breakthrough spotting, moodiness, cramping, breast tenderness, fluid retention, nausea, or headaches. Also, over the counter progesterone creams may not achieve high enough blood levels to oppose any particular prescription estrogen, and thereby increase chances of endometrial malignancy and or uterine hyperplasia (buildup of the uterine lining). Prescription HT and over the counter hormonal creams should never be used together.

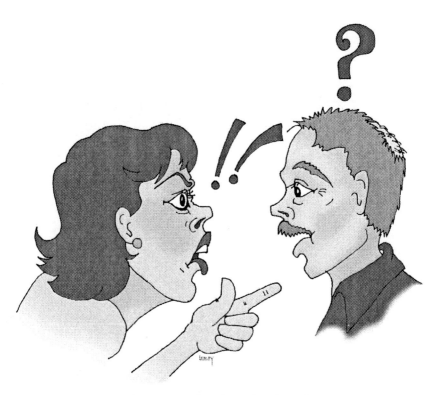

When your husband asks why?
And then you tell him off!

Chapter 4:

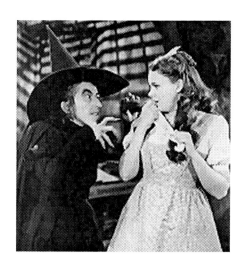

Hormone Replacement Therapy & The 2002 Women's Health Initiative Study: Why Is There So Much Confusion? (Including 2006 Update)

By Neil C. Boland, M.D., F.A.C.O.G.

Ding, Dong, The Wicked Witch Is Dead

As baby boomers, most of us can recall exactly what we were doing on November 22, 1963 when we discovered that President John F. Kennedy had been assassinated. Similarly, I too have vivid flashbacks of a late afternoon on July 10, 2002 when I returned to my office after an emergency cesarean section at the hospital. I only been gone for less than two hours, and I remember distinctly over 20 charts quickly appeared on my desk, which were not there when I left. Almost all of these messages were from anxious patients requesting telephone callbacks. Unknown to me then, the news was out. The many years I had spent carefully documenting potential health benefits and risks of hormonal therapy (HT) for each one of my menopausal patients had become abruptly irrelevant.

Newspaper and television media had suddenly and proclaimed that day that use of hormonal therapy was "dangerous". Little or no other unbiased information was given. Women taking hormones should check with their physician about what specific course of action they should take. Many did. Some didn't, and just discarded their medication. Almost immediately, many of them experienced the worst month of their lives. Menopausal symptoms dominated and debilitated their lives. On the one hand, the media were scaring them to death if they continued to take HT, and now they found their lives unbearable. My office practice was swamped for months by a never ending deluge of ill-feeling irritable dysphoric patients requiring emergency consultation.

Doctor, what should I do? Doctor, aren't you keeping up? Doctor, what do you mean you haven't seen the published study yet? (It hadn't been yet.)

Unfortunately, the Women's Health Initiative (WHI) Study would not actually be published until a week later on July 17, 2002 in JAMA, the Journal of the American Medical Association. It was thought at that point in time this study would radically change the practice of menopausal medicine as we know it. Incoming calls from terrified patients overloaded our office phone lines for days and weeks to come. Unbelievably, almost no physician in the United States had had prior access to the study, much less had analyzed it beforehand. Much like 9/11/2001, chaos and confusion were rampant.

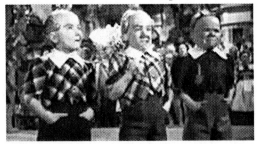

The Munchkins danced and sang joyfully over and over. The wicked witch was finally dead. Little did anyone realize at that time they had instead wounded Glenda the Good Witch of The West. After all, friendly fire can be just as deadly as enemy fire.

The Background: Women's Health Initiative Study

What set the stage for this series of events? In 1942, the FDA approved a hormonal medication called Premarin to help alleviate menopausal hot flashes. It was amazingly effective. Later in the 1960s, synthetic hormones were developed in the form of oral contraceptive pills (OCPs) to prevent pregnancy. For the first time, women found it was effective and convenient to use hormonal therapy, allowing them control of the timing of pregnancies. For most of them, OCPs also significantly improved problems with heavy or prolonged menstrual flow and painful periods. The introduction of new lower dose OCPs over the next several decades afforded reductions in side effects, improved safety, and better compliance.

But the mid-1970s, it was discovered that higher rates of endometrial cancer (uterine lining) were detected in those patients taking estrogen only. The addition of progestins (progesterone hormones) to the estrogen seemed to mimic the natural hormonal milieu interaction in the pre-menopausal woman, and actually reduced the incidence of this cancer below a control group, thereby actually preventing cancer.

The progestins unfortunately were noted to increase the side effects of moodiness, breakthrough bleeding, and feeling bloated. Various cyclic regimens of taking hormones were formulated. Some regimens required taking estrogen for certain number of days a month, and the progestin was added only on certain days in order to generate a controlled withdrawal bleed (period). While this was effective over time in reducing breakthrough spotting, many women objected to these monthly periods. Because of this, various *continuous* HRT regimens were formulated, meaning that the same combination of estrogen and progestin are taken daily, which essentially eliminated periods altogether for the vast majority of patients, making them very content.

Hormonal therapy dramatically improved the quality of life (QOL) of virtually all of these women. Hot flashes, night sweats, insomnia, vaginal dryness, painful intercourse, irritability, mood swings, and difficulties in concentration all improved. Rates of osteoporosis dropped as well as it was discovered HT improved bone density and reduced fracture risk. It was even postulated that HT might even reduce their risk of development of atherosclerosis (hardening of the arteries), and thereby subsequently reduce their risk of heart attack and stroke. After all, it was true that women who had had their ovaries removed surgically at young ages appeared to have higher risk profiles for heart disease. Also, it was also postulated that the estrogen deficiency of menopause might actually trigger atherosclerosis as well.

In the early 1990s, the National Institute of Health (NIH), a highly respected U.S. governmental department for medical research, decided to initiate the multi-million dollar WHI study. This study, which terminated its second arm in March 2004, involved over 161,000 women, from age 50-79. They were geographically well distributed all across the United States with data gathered by respected medical centers. The subjects were followed over 15 years in a prospective randomized double-blind controlled fashion to evaluate objectively the long term risks and benefits of hormone therapy in disease prevention. It is felt that this type of scientific study is the gold standard of investigation. The study was done from a specific point in time in going forward into the future, in which random selections of patients are made, and neither the patient nor investigator involved really knew which medication the patient was taking.

The WHI Study was one of the largest, most highly respected, well done scientific endeavors ever undertaken. It included 1) estrogen plus progestin and 2) estrogen only hormone therapies. Areas studied for disease prevention included evaluation of rates of female breast and colorectal cancer, heart attack, stroke, blood clot formation, and hip fracture in patients in both categories of hormone replacement noted above. Further derivative studies evaluated quality of life, cognitive function, diabetes, peripheral arterial disease, and specific gynecologic malignancies. Other observational studies included evaluation of calcium and Vitamin D, dietary programs, and urinary incontinence.

The Women's Health Initiative Study was designed to start in 1993 to test the safety of two major hormonal medications manufactured by the Wyeth-Ayerst pharmaceutical company. These are: Premarin (0.625 mg Conjugated Equine Estrogens, also known as CEE), and Prempro (0.625 mg. CEE combined with 2.5 mg. Medroxyprogesterone Acetate, also known as MPA). Premarin is an estrogen only derivative of pregnant mare urine. (No, the mares are *not* mistreated as special interest group rumors would lead you to believe).

Prempro is a combination of estrogen and progestin. In one arm of the study, 16,000 women with a uterus were randomized to receive either Prempro or a placebo (sugar) pill. The other 10,000 women who had already had hysterectomy received either Premarin or placebo. Please keep in mind that no other hormonal medications besides Premarin and Prempro were studied in the WHI, even if they were already FDA-approved in 1993 or before.

In addition, Wyeth-Ayerst also sponsored a trial of HT, known as the HERS trial (the Heart and Estrogen/ Progestin Replacement Study). The goal of this important study was to determine if the theory of so-called "secondary prevention" of coronary vascular disease was a valid one. In other words, do Premarin and Prempro prevent heart attacks among those patients who have already suffered a heart attack, and/or exhibit symptoms of severe angina?

In 1998, the findings of the study surprised most investigators. In this selected group of patients with pre-existing cardiovascular disease, and the rate of heart attack, decreased slightly over a five-year time span. However, it was found that HT actually *increased* the rate of heart attacks in the first year of taking the medication. Immediately, the American Heart Association (AHA) recommended that hormonal therapy *not be initiated for prevention of a second heart attack among women who already had pre-existing cardiovascular disease. The AHA also recommended that it was medically acceptable to continue HT in those patients already taking the medication and doing fine on, whether they had pre-existing vascular disease or not.*

The Women's Health Initiative study was also ongoing during the HERS study. The WHI had an automatic built-in study termination condition that if important findings were uncovered that were statistically significant, that certain study arms could be stopped. The WHI safety monitoring board then recommended stopping part of study in 2002 which was scheduled to end three years later in 2005. It was felt that the incidence of breast cancer in the study population was slightly increased in the Prempro population compared to controls. This important news was somehow leaked to the press, and prematurely released as front-page headlines in most newspapers across the USA.

WHI: Garbage In, Garbage Out?

Finally, a week later on July 17, 2002, the Journal of the American Medical Association published the WHI Study. Immediately, this landmark study was carefully read and reread by thousands of researchers, academicians, physicians, and other health care providers the world over. This study was exceptionally well designed and well executed, and has demonstrated that hormonal therapy is, in general, not appropriate for use in "secondary prevention" of certain disease processes (the disease already exists, and can we prevent it or slow its evolution)? What about "primary prevention" (prevent the disease before it develops)? We simply do not yet know. Was the entire population of women studied a truly representative sample of menopausal women as a whole? No, it was not, and the danger lies in applying its findings to menopausal women of all ages.

Chances are overwhelmingly good that if your health care provider has done his or her homework, is well trained, and has critically analyzed past and current literature, they have already come to the same conclusions we have. Our opinion about the WHI being flawed is widespread among most well trained up to date doctors today. The study findings are NOT universally applicable to *all* menopausal women. This is not really as controversial as you might be led to believe by the media. What mystifies physicians is why their voices seem to have so little credibility among the public.

Why is there this credibility gap? The lay press, print, and television are not physicians. Media incomes are under massive assault from the Internet, where gargantuan amounts of information in the 21st century move at light speed. Classified advertising revenue has plummeted due to massive changes in societal behavior, such as usage of Ebay and Craig's List for buying and selling. The media stand to loose literally billions if they cannot keep their readers' attention. The best way to do this is what they seem to do well.......create controversy where none really exists. Keep the public confused and scared. Try to connect the dots of cause and effect by mere speculation, and forget scientific investigation and rationality.

This is the definition of junk media. Unfortunately for society, this is the perfect setup for plaintiff attorney junk litigation and internet snake oil salesmen. Personally, I don't mind controversy in politics, religion, or theories of evolution, but I DO MIND when controversy seems to generate behavior detrimental to the health and welfare of our women.

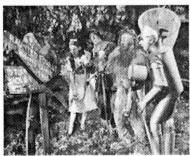

Now let's carefully examine the characteristics of the WHI Study Population:

WHI
Baseline Characteristics

Characteristic	HRT group n= 8,505	Placebo n=8,102
Age at Screening	63.2 yr.	63.3 yr.
Prior Use Hormones	26.1 %	25.6%
Body Mass Index (kg/m2)	28.5	28.5
Never Smokers	49.6%	50.0%
Diabetes	4.4%	4.4%
Hypertension	35.7%	36.4%
Statin Use at Screening	6.9%	6.8%
Family Hx Breast Cancer	16%	15.3%
History of Heart Attack	1.6%	1.9%
History of Cardiac Bypass/PTCA	1.1%	1.5%

Reprinted from the Writing Group for the Women's Health Initiative Investigators. JAMA. 288: 321-333, 2002.

Why is the WHI study population as noted above not indicative of menopausal women in general? As noted in previous chapters, the average age of menopause is currently 51.7 years, which is quite younger than the much older average hypothetical 63 year old patient analyzed in WHI. Remember menopausal symptoms seem to start much earlier than this, generally in the mid-forties. Does this really make a difference? Of course it does.

The Typical of WHI Patient Age

Is a thirty year old postmenopausal patient who has undergone surgical menopause for symptomatic pelvic endometriosis different from the 63 year old hypothetical patient who has undergone spontaneous menopause? The 30 year old patient has *not* undergone as much slow deleterious plaque accumulation inside her arterial walls as the average 63 year old study patient has. Would this make a difference in her comparative risk profile for stroke and heart attack? It makes intuitive sense to all of us that a woman's body is much different at ages 30, 40, 50, 60 and so on. Ask any woman. In fact, now four years after the initial WHI publication, most of menopausal research in this category is now beginning to recognize that hormonal therapy likely has differential effects in different ages, disease processes, cardiovascular risk profiles, and neurochemical imbalances (read more about this in subsequent chapters).

Obesity

Researchers used a calculation called body mass index (BMI) in order to quantify a subject's weight. The upper limit of normal BMI is 25 kilograms per meter squared of body surface area, with about 18-25 being normal range, 25-30 being overweight, and any patient with a BMI higher than 30 is obese. The average subject's BMI of 28.5 was in the overweight category, and automatically places that patient in a higher risk cardiovascular profile. A BMI of 28.5 means the average subject was 5'5" tall and weighed 170 pounds! While we as Americans have tended to become more sedentary and obese as we grow older, is this truly a representative example of all postmenopausal women?

Other Important Risk Factors

About half the study population were either current smokers or former smokers. Over one third of them had hypertension, and about 7% were on cholesterol-lowering medications. Between 1- 2% of the study population had either had cardiac bypass surgery or a prior heart attack. Therefore, in many ways, the WHI population were older, more obese, sicker, and had much poorer cardiovascular risk profiles than typical women going through menopause.

The real fallacy in acceptance of the WHI findings on face value has not so much to do with the findings themselves, which are indeed valid for the special population that was studied. However, there is faulty scientific validity of extrapolating or applying the study data to all menopausal women of all ages. Menopause is much more complicated than that. Even more importantly, a women's quality-of-life has to be taken into consideration somewhere in this decision. It is obvious that the WHI did not study women actually going through the menopause.

Who Ya Gonna Call?

We have established the type of menopausal patient analyzed in the WHI. However, we as gynecologists and menopausal medicine specialists seldom see the typical WHI patient: the 63 year old, 5 foot five, 170 pound, obese female with multiple cardiovascular risk factors, requesting consideration for *initiation* of hormonal therapy for hot flashes. Of course we would take this patient off hormones immediately if she is already taking them.

Much more commonly, we see the perimenopausal or menopausal non-smoking or never smoked 48-year-old, who is 5'7" tall and weighs 145 pounds, with minimal medical problems, has normal cholesterol and blood pressure readings, who reports her quality-of-life is horrible. She does monthly self breast exams, and exercises regularly. She reports significant daily work impairment, generated by lack of sleep, hot flashes, night sweats, mood alterations, and an inability to concentrate. She is terrified of breast cancer, and has delayed her visit to the doctor thinking that her condition is unusual because it is persisted longer than two years. She went off birth-control pills six years ago, because her husband got a vasectomy.

Should we as clinicians treat both categories of patients identically? *The answer is a resounding NO!* Just as the earlier patient, the latter patient should be given a full medical history, physical exam, blood work, mammogram, and bone density evaluation. She should have a full informed consent discussion of the pros, cons, and side effects of hormonal therapy. She may choose to try CAHM (Complimentary, Alternative, or Homeopathic Medications), hormonal therapy, other prescription medications which may help, or simply continue to suffer. If she chooses to take hormonal therapy, she should be made aware that hormonal therapy is not a lifelong commitment, but should be given at the lowest dose as possible for the shortest length of time. For any questions or problems, telephone support should be available, and close follow-up is advised.

The WHI Study Findings: Estrogen and Progestin Arm

As outlined above, the WHI profile patient studied who is seeking to *initiate hormonal therapy is not as common as one would be led to believe. However, the WHI showed what would occur in these 16,000 patients.*

E+P HT Adverse Effects:

Only 2.5% of women in the estrogen plus progestin study had these health events. These results tell us that during one year, <u>for every 10,000 women taking estrogen plus progestin, we would expect</u>:

- 8 more women with breast cancer (0.08% higher risk). In other words, 38 women taking estrogen plus progestin would have breast cancer compared with 30 women taking placebo. Eight patients in 10,000 is 0.08% higher frequency, which is a ridiculously small increase. After four years of therapy, a small increase in invasive breast cancer was noted.

- 7 more women with heart attacks (0.07% higher risk). In other words, 37 women taking estrogen plus progestin would have heart attacks compared to 30 women taking placebo. Seven patients in 10,000 is 0.07% higher frequency, which is a ridiculously small increase.

- 8 more women with strokes (0.08% higher risk as above)

- 18 more women with blood clots or venous thrombotic events (thrombophlebitis or pulmonary embolism) (0.18% higher risk as above)

E+P HT Beneficial Effects

These results also suggest that for every 10,000 women taking estrogen plus progestin, we would expect:

- 6 fewer colorectal cancers (0.06% lower risk)

- 5 fewer hip fractures (0.05% lower risk) with fewer in other bones

E+P HT Neutral Effects

Slightly lower risks of endometrial cancer and overall death rates due to other causes in those in the estrogen/ progestin group were noted.

In summary, then, more women taking estrogen plus progestin had a serious health event than did women taking place, but the adverse results are ridiculously small. Statistical significance was achieved only with heart attacks, strokes, and venous thrombotic events.

Adverse and Beneficial Risks of Estrogen/ Progestin
Treatment per 10,000 Patients

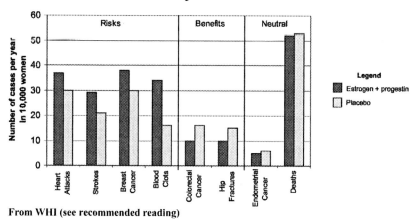

From WHI (see recommended reading)

From WHI (see recommended reading)

The WHI Study Findings: Estrogen Only Arm

In March 2004, the WHI ended its estrogen only arm, which had continued approximately 2 years beyond the estrogen and progestin arm of the study. The results demonstrated some surprising similarities and differences with the previously published results.

These results show said during one year, for every 10,000 women taking estrogen only (as designated by CEE) , we would expect:

Estrogen Only Adverse Events

- 12 more women with strokes

- 6 more women with venous thrombotic events (WHI says uncertain)

- 1 more woman with colorectal cancer (WHI says neutral)

Estrogen Only HT Benefits

- 6 *fewer* women with hip fractures.

- 7 *fewer* women with breast cancer (WHI says uncertain)

- 4 *fewer heart attacks (WHI says neutral)*

In summary, taking into account all of the diseases studied during 6.8 years of follow-up in patients taking Estrogen only:

1) The increased risk of stroke and the decreased risk of fractures we now see in women taking estrogen alone are similar to the effects of estrogen plus progestin.

2) The findings that estrogen only did not increase breast cancers or decrease colorectal cancers were different from the estrogen plus progestin.

Adverse and Beneficial Effects of Estrogen Only

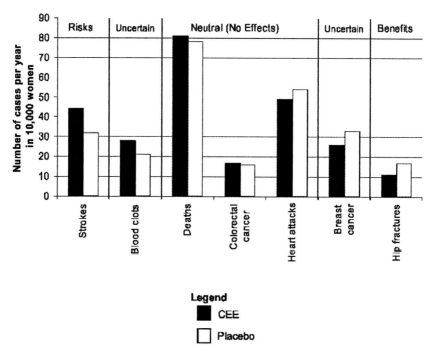

Commentary on the WHI 2002 Results

It is very important to mention that I frequently mention to patients taking estrogen only without progestin that we still have no evidence that taking estrogen by itself increases breast cancer, which seems to be a major fear of some patients. In fact, there is a suggestion when from this latest WHI data above that conjugated equine estrogens may actually *slightly reduce* breast cancer risk below a control population. Keep in mind that not all estrogens on the market are conjugated equine estrogens (CEE), and the vast majority of others commercially available have not yet been studied.

A second point is that relative to breast cancer, the differences between the two study groups may implicate the progestin component of Prempro, called Provera (medroxyprogesterone acetate), as the culprit.

However, no studies have yet been done to confirm or disprove this hypothesis.

A third point is that as I write this chapter, it is overwhelming to me the extremely small number of patients per year that may be involved with these disease processes. We are, in worst case scenario, discussing a fraction of a 1% increased risk, except for stroke and thrombophlebitis, which are slightly higher. It is imperative that the clinician communicate these small risks to the patient so that she may make an informed choice.

✑ ✑ ✑

Important Updates On New WHI Findings since 2002:

Cognitive Function: (JAMA, 289: No. 20. May 28, 2003)

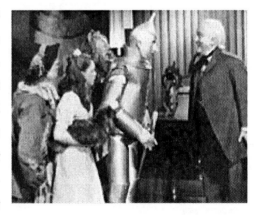

The Women's Health Initiative Memory Study, also known as WHIMS, has been finished, relative to the use of estrogen and progestin and to estrogen only. This was a study of over 4,500 participants aged 65-79, evaluated relative to their cognitive function, mild cognitive decline, and dementia. The findings were that estrogen and progestin do not protect women from mild cognitive declines, compared with placebo. In addition, the medication increases the chance of more severe dementia, but only for women age 65 and over. This translates into only 23 out of every 10,000 patients for the combined medication and 28 out of every 10,000 patients for estrogen only. This means an increased risk of 0.0023%, and 0.0028% respectively for the two groups, which is very tiny indeed. Further follow-up is being performed on these patients to determine if cognitive impairment continues after the medication has been terminated.

~~~ ~~~ ~~~

Breast Cancer: (JAMA, 289: No. 24, June 25, 2003)

This was a continued follow up of the original WHI patients on combined estrogen and progestin therapy. There was a continued finding of 8 additional cases of breast cancer for every 10,000 patients studied. In addition, the breast cancers appear to be more invasive and larger at discovery than in the placebo group. There was a higher incidence of abnormal mammograms in the study patient group after hormonal therapy had been discontinued. This was likely due to the increased radiographic density of the breast generated from HT.

An additional analysis study of estrogen only patients (JAMA, 295: No. 14, April, 2006) was just published in April, 2006. This study demonstrated a continued 23% *reduction in breast cancer* after approximately 7 years of follow-up, which was non-statistically significant. Reduction in breast cancer risk was generally seen in two specific types of breast cancer, namely ductal carcinoma and in early-stage disease. Estrogen only therapy appeared to lower breast cancer risk in lower risk individuals, and elevate it in higher risk individuals.

~~~ ~~~ ~~~

Stroke: (JAMA, 289: No. 20, May 28, 2003)

This was a continued follow up study also of the original WHI patients on combined estrogen and progestin therapy. There was a continued finding of seven additional strokes per 10,000 patients in the study group, relative to placebo (1.8% versus 1.3%). Most of the strokes involved were of the thrombotic variety (blood clot in the brain). The incidence of hemorrhagic stroke (bleeding inside the brain) was not affected. The authors suggest that three risk factors which can be altered in stroke prevention are smoking cessation, controlling blood pressure, and vitamin C supplementation.

ℰℑ ℰℑ ℰℑ

Venous Thrombosis: (JAMA, 292: No. 13, October 6, 2004)

This continued WHI follow up study continued to demonstrate 18 additional strokes per 10,000 women per year after an average 5.6 years follow up. The major risk factors for thrombosis in this group appeared to be obesity and factor V Leiden deficiency. Factor Leiden V deficiency is found in about 5% of the American population, associated primarily with European descent. It is the most common genetic deficiency associated with venous thrombosis. This genetic mutation affords a five times higher risk of thrombosis than the general population. However, most patients with this mutation will never have a thrombotic event. The use of aspirin for this study group of estrogen and progestin patients did not lower the risk of venous thrombosis.

ℰℑ ℰℑ ℰℑ

Bone Density: (JAMA, 290: No.1, October 13, 2003)

In the WHI study population taking estrogen and progestin therapy, after an average of 5.6 years follow-up, there was a 24% reduction in all fractures and a 33% reduction in hip fractures. Hip bone density increased 3.7% in the study group compared to 0.13% in the placebo group. A WHI concluded that estrogen and progestin therapy should not be recommended as first-line treatment for prevention of osteoporosis due to other overall potential risks.

ℰℑ ℰℑ ℰℑ

<u>Diabetes:</u> (Diabetologia, July, 2004)

After an average of 5.6 years of follow-up WHI researchers concluded that estrogen and progestin therapy reduced the risk of newly treated diabetes by 21%. Only 3.5% of the study population became diabetic during this time compared with 4.2% of the placebo group. It appears that hormonal therapy patients actually showed a decrease in blood sugar and insulin levels, as well as decreasing weight and waist size. It was felt that these findings may be so significant that the study should be redone in future postmenopausal hormonal trials.

❧ ❧ ❧

<u>Colorectal Cancer:</u> (NEJM, Vol. 350: p. 991-1004, March 4, 2004)

The WHI population taking estrogen and progestin therapy after an average 5.6 years of continued follow-up yielded a 44% decrease in colorectal malignancy. The histologic type of malignancy was with similar in both groups. However, it was noted in the study population taking hormonal therapy that the malignancies encountered were of more advanced staging (more distant spread and metastases) in 76% versus 39% in the placebo group.

❧ ❧ ❧

<u>Heart Disease:</u> (NEJM, 349: 523-534, August 7, 2003)

Further analysis of estrogen plus progestin (E+P) patients was performed. Combined therapy does not protect the heart and may even increase the risk of CHD (Coronary Heart Disease) in generally healthy postmenopausal women. Overall, there was a 24% higher risk of CHD among women in the E+P study compared to women taking placebo (6 extra cases of CHD per 10,000 women per year). The greater risk of CHD was highest during the first year after starting hormone therapy (an 81% increase). E+P had no major effect on the risk of angina, coronary bypass surgery, angioplasty, or congestive heart failure.

A second very recent 2006 article was published regarding the use of estrogen only in the WHI population (Archives of Internal Medicine, 166: No. 3, February 13, 2006). The original study was stopped ahead of schedule in February 2004 by the NIH because of increased stroke risk. During 7.1 years of follow up, estrogen provided no overall protection against heart attack or coronary death in generally healthy postmenopausal women most of whom were more than 10 years past menopause when they entered the study. However, in women ages 50-59 years of age at study entry (3,110 patients), there was enough data to show that after 7 years these younger women were no more likely to have a heart attack than placebo, and in fact were 37% less likely to occur.

ლ ლ ლ

Vitamin D and Calcium Supplementation: (NEJM: 354:669-683, February 16, 2006)

WHI investigators also performed the WHI Calcium and Vitamin D Study, providing 7 years of follow-up data for over 36,000 patients compared with placebo. This study was the largest randomized trial ever done on this subject. They found that calcium plus vitamin D supplements improved hip bone density compared to placebo and lowered the risk of hip fractures in some groups, but did not reduce fracture risk in all groups. It did increase kidney stones, and did not reduce risk of colorectal cancer. The current national recommendations say that women over 50 years should have daily total calcium intakes of 1000-1200 mg/day and vitamin D intakes in the range of 400-600 IU.

Among women 60 years of age and older, those assigned to active calcium and Vitamin D supplementation daily had a 21% decreased risk of hip fracture compared to women 60 and over who were taking placebo (17 compared to 23 cases per 10,000 women each year). This difference was statistically significant.

ളി ളി ളി

Urinary Incontinence: (JAMA, 293: No. 8, February 23, 2005)

Women who did not have urinary incontinence when they joined the WHI study had an increased risk of developing any type of incontinence after 1 year if they were in the active hormone group compared to the placebo group. This risk was 39% higher for women taking active hormones in the E+P trial compared to those taking placebo. The risk was 52% higher for women taking active hormones in the estrogen only group compared to placebo. The risk was highest for developing stress incontinence, followed by mixed incontinence.

Among women who reported incontinence when they joined the WHI, the active hormones in both the E+P and estrogen only trials worsened both the frequency and amount of incontinence after one year, compared to placebo. In addition, women taking the active hormones were more likely than women taking placebo to report that their incontinence bothered or disturbed them and that it limited their daily activities.

The researchers concluded that postmenopausal hormone therapy should not be prescribed to prevent or treat urinary incontinence.

ളി ളി ളി

Other Gynecologic Malignancies: (JAMA: 290: No. 13, October 1, 2003)

The WHI investigators showed a 19% decrease in the rate of endometrial (uterine) cancer in the estrogen and progestin group, as expected, as compared to placebo. Thus, women taking E+P have a risk of endometrial cancer that is similar to or slightly less than women taking placebo. Progestin appears to cancel beneficially the harmful effect of estrogen in the uterus, as previous studies showed.

The tiny increase in ovarian cancer is consistent with reports from observational studies of estrogen alone and some other forms of combined hormones. However, the number of ovarian cancers in WHI was small (only 32), so it is possible that this was just a chance finding, and likely was just chance. No other study has linked this particular hormone combination with an increased risk of ovarian cancer. In women taking placebo, the rate of ovarian cancer would be 27 cancers per 100,000 (which is only 2.7 per 10,000) women per year. In women taking E+P, the rate would be 42 cancers per 100,000 (which is only 4.2 per 10,000 women per year, an increase of 1.5. Even if this effect of E+P is real and not a chance finding, ovarian cancer remains a very rare disease in women taking these hormones.

The numbers of other gynecologic cancers (cancers of the cervix, fallopian tube, and peritoneum) were so small, it was not possible to draw conclusions about the effects of combined hormone use on these cancers, but it is extremely unlikely a relationship exists.

℘ ℘ ℘

Quality of Life (NEJM, May 18, 2003)

WHI randomization of estrogen plus progestin (HT) therapy was done in over 1,100 patients age 50-79, with mean age 63. HT resulted in no significant effects on general health, vitality, mental health, depressive symptoms, or sexual satisfaction. The use of estrogen plus progestin was associated with a statistically significant but small and not clinically meaningful benefit in terms of sleep disturbance, physical functioning, and bodily pain after one year. At three years, there were no significant benefits in terms of any quality-of-life outcomes.

Among women 50 to 54 years of age with moderate-to-severe vasomotor symptoms at base line, estrogen and progestin improved vasomotor symptoms and resulted in a small benefit in terms of sleep disturbance but no benefit in terms of the other quality-of-life outcomes. In this trial in postmenopausal women, estrogen plus progestin did *not* have a clinically meaningful effect on health-related quality of life.

My reaction to this study is that it very misleading to generalize these findings to all menopausal women. Women with an average age of 63 (or older) are too old to be a representative example of the typical symptomatic menopausal patient. Therefore, this study (just like the rest of the WHI findings) has to be carefully interpreted. We have already commented earlier in this chapter that the WHI population is *not* the group of women beating our door down to seek help with hot flashes. HT may have minimal positive effects on the average WHI patient (an older subset of patients). However, in contrast, the *average* symptomatic postmenopausal patient is younger physiologically and perhaps chronologically, forming a completely different group of patients for which HT is miraculously effective.

❧ ❧ ❧

Quality of Life, Continued (JAMA, 294: No. 2, July 13, 2005)

The data analysis of this WHI study focused on symptoms such as hot flashes, night sweats, vaginal dryness, and pain or stiffness. Findings:

- Women who had menopausal symptoms when they joined the WHI, regardless of their age, were more likely to have these symptoms after stopping study pills than women who did not have symptoms.

- After stopping their study pills, women in the active hormone group reported more symptoms than women in the placebo pill group.

- Women who took hormones before they joined the WHI were more likely to have hot flashes or night sweats after stopping than women who did not take hormones.

- Women tried to manage their symptoms in different ways, including drinking more fluids, exercising, and talking with a health care provider. Most women found these efforts helpful.

- Compared with women who tried other strategies to help with symptoms, fewer women who tried herbal or natural hormones said they helped.

- Very few women started prescription hormones after stopping their study pills.

These findings answer some questions about what happens when hormone therapy is stopped. Women who are thinking about taking hormones for menopausal symptoms should keep in mind that they may have these symptoms again after stopping.

℘ ℘ ℘

Lung Cancer: (Cancer Research, University of Pittsburgh Cancer Institute Publication, February 15, 2005)

Although the WHI did not study or address lung cancer, I have to mention fascinating current ongoing research on the relationship of estrogen and lung cancer. Lung cancer is the number one cancer killer of women, killing about 60,000 women in the U.S. each year. (In second place is colon cancer, and third is breast cancer).

Non-small cell lung cancer comprises 80 percent of lung cancer cases. Some population studies have suggested that women develop the disease at an earlier age and with less reported tobacco exposure than men, prompting scientists to search for biological reasons that could account for these discrepancies. Investigations by Dr. Jill Siegfried and others have indicated that lung cancer is different in women than in men, both with regard to the type of tumors that develop and the molecular mechanisms underlying the disease.

Since women have higher circulating estrogen levels than men, blocking estrogen receptors with new drugs in lung cancer cells could prove beneficial in preventing lung cancer in women at high risk, much like blocking estrogen's effect has been shown to reduce breast cancer risk.

This study looked at two common estrogen receptors (ER alpha and ER beta) on lung cancer cell lines, cultured normal lung cells and normal and tumor tissues from lung cancer patients. The researchers found that *normal* lung tissue rarely showed detectable levels of ER alpha, whereas *lung tumor cells* had significantly higher levels of this receptor. ER beta was found in both normal and tumor cells. Treating cultured lung cancer cells with estrogen resulted in increased cell division. Estrogen given to animals with human lung cancers resulted in increased tumor growth. Anti-estrogens inhibited this effect. All these results suggest that estrogen may play a role in lung cancer development, much as it does in breast cancer.

Previous work by Dr. Siegfried has shown a gene for the protein gastrin-releasing peptide receptor, or GRPR, also is more active in lung tissues in women than in men, again providing a biological reason for why lung cancer differs between the sexes.

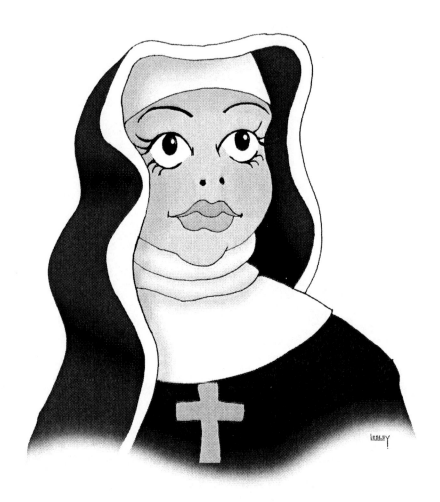

Thrill of romance?
I could be a nun in a convent!

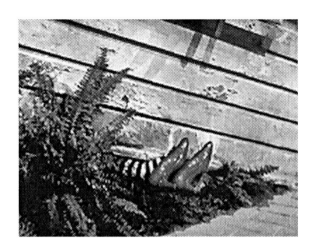

Chapter 5:

The Menopause And Your Sexuality: Older CAN Be Better!

By Neil C. Boland, M.D., F.A.C.O.G.

Introduction
by Linda LaVelle, ATIE, ITEC

Okay, so it is 9:00 p.m. and you are ready to go to bed and dream of having a good nights sleep. Then along comes the movement! The legs wrap around your torso, the hand comes around your breasts, and the kisses come around your neck area, you are thinking of a good nights sleep, and he is thinking of a moment in sex heaven! You don't want to disappoint him but you want to go to bed, and really sex was not on your #1 list of things to do tonight! It drives you crazy, yet you feel guilty because you know that his sexual urge is by far greater than yours right now and you don't know what to do except sleep is calling you and you turn around and tell him that you are really tired from the hectic day. Whew! Another night to just rest and recuperate... maybe tomorrow will be better than how you feel right now!

You see, you are lacking one big thing and that is the hormone testosterone! Without this hormone, you could be a nun for the rest of your life. You could easily live in a world without sex, and it would not bother you in the least! Don't feel guilty because that is what menopause does to you. If we did not have hormone therapy, we could all go to a monastery and become nuns or just become celibate! It would not bother me in the least, except that I have a partner that is waiting on my beck and call and wants sex more frequently than I do! I get in the mood. I become a tart, as the English say, and I put myself into another frame of mind! I become the woman he met and fell in love with.

You see, I am a woman in menopause and things are different now. I don't want you to feel bad, and I don't want you to feel sorry for me, as I have a wonderful and fulfilling life, but it is just different from what I envisioned. I feel very sexy and smarter. I have ideas that would never have entered my brain at the age of 35 or 40. I wish that I could have the body of a 35 year old woman, and still keep the brains of a 50 year old! What a powerhouse she would be! I am lacking one thing however, and that is the sexual drive that I had in my 30's and 40's. I don't feel as if I am missing anything, as I am in another era right now, and that is the searching for what is life really all about, and how can I achieve quality of life?

Sexuality seems to take a second seat to this question, and that seems to be the reason why some men may start searching for a younger woman. Their sexuality peaks at a different time than women, and they still want sex frequently, whereas we are slowing down on the frequency, and we just want more quality time... Don't get me wrong, because we still like to go shopping for intimate things and to look sexy. We just don't want the wild thing as much as our better half wants it, and that is perfectly alright with us! So what is wrong with this picture, and what can we do to make our lives more productive and fulfilling? I ask this question of my gynecologist and co-author, how can a woman get back her sexuality that she had when she was 35 or 40?

Dr. Boland:

Linda, I think you outlined the problem perfectly that we gynecologists encounter each and every day. It's the discordant sexual mindset of the average 55 year old menopausal patient and her say, for example, 55-60 year old husband. It's a frequent office complaint. Probably the two most difficult problems we encounter in the older patient: Doctor, what can I do to loose weight, and what can you do to improve my sex drive (libido)? (BTW, my partner wanted me to ask you.)

First, the news is not all bad. The sexually active older patient does have some *advantages* over the younger patient. I have observed the older patient is often much more emotionally and intellectually mature, confident, experienced, and realistic about herself, and about what she can and cannot accomplish. She no longer is burdened with menstrual problems such as vaginal bleeding, and menstrual pain. The fear of becoming pregnant is gone. She has become more focused on her health, because Mother Nature makes her do it and calls it to her attention in a myriad of ways. She begins to focus a little more on her mortality and where she fits into the grand overall scheme of humanity. By age 50 or so, the children are leaving the nest, and she has more time for herself . (For working women, this may or not be true). She perhaps has a little more "ME" time, and some studies show this can be one of the *happiest* times of her lives. Some women have a refocused spiritualism relative to their faiths. They begin exercise programs, loose weight, and adopt new hobbies or skills as their schedules allow. Often, she has more financial resources available than she did when she was younger. She and her partner can now travel to those faraway romantic places they have always dreamed about. (In Florida, we just plan our next exit strategies for the next hurricane!) So the news is not all bad!

Doctors label the problem of poor libido in both sexes as Hypoactive Sexual Desire Disorder (also called HSDD). Estrogen and testosterone deficiencies both contribute to the problem and have a negative impact on female sexual function. HSDD affects at least one third of all women that are peri- or post-menopausal. Compounding this problem can be severe stress, anxiety, relationship conflict, self image and self esteem changes, as well as overall medical problems. Medications frequently have a profound effect in lowering sex drive in both sexes.

Being around the fairer sex all day, it has always been astounding to me the differences in mindsets between the sexes. How does this problem begin anyway? It's important to outline. Mature women as well as younger ones have multiple layers of complexity in their sexuality to begin with, and their control panels consist of dials, switches, levers, and icons. Men have only one switch: It's a toggle switch: Off or On.

Both men and women can have sexual dysfunction, but this book is not about men. Women's switches tend to be more layered:

- First Layer: It's the relationship, Stupid (I said that for the *men, not the women, because women already know this!). Men need the education. Some men are not nearly as focused on this issue as women. Men's evolutionary wiring and testosterone driven gonads tend to be the bus driver; whereas in women, it's usually emotional intimacy that is the goal.*

- Second Layer: Women tend to be somewhat more burdened with psychologic distractions than men. Little Melinda and Jeffrey are in the next room are trying to sleep....so be quiet! Anxiety, depression, stress, fatigue, money problems, and family issues can be a third partner in bed. Prior traumatic experiences, mood disturbances, and illicit drug and alcohol abuse can also interfere. And as we all know, if mama ain't happy, ain't nobody happy!

- Third Layer: Health problems, such as the endocrine deficiencies of estrogen and testosterone can not only create HSDD, but if untreated, can lead to very painful intercourse due to a very thin and dry vaginal lining. Pain causes avoidance behavior. This can add a further mental aversional hurdle of negative feedback to the woman's experience. Orthopedic problems and other multiple medical problems can contribute as well.

- Fourth Layer: Medications, such as SSRI anti-depressants (for example Prozac or Zoloft) and a host of others can inhibit sex drive.

Relative to the third layer of medical problems, HSDD is defined as the persistent or recurrent deficiency or absence of sexual fantasies, or the desire for sexual activity, accompanied by personal distress or interpersonal difficulty. Unfortunately, this absence of desire is strongly correlated with low feelings of happiness and low self esteem. Although low libido can occur at any age with interference at any at the layers outlined above in both men and women, the menopausal woman is at particular risk for HSDD.

Dr. Phil Sarrell has studied this issue and has reported that at least 40% of women in a menopausal clinic experienced low sexual desire, and at least 30-50 % of women who have had their ovaries removed report reduced desire. It has been long hypothesized that hormonal deficiencies contribute to HSDD, with low estrogen and especially testosterone. Other potential endocrine problems are those of adrenal deficiency, depression, and thyroid disease.

Estrogen levels plummet steeply in the first year after menopause, and continue to decline over time to at least 50% lower than women who are capable of reproducing. This low estrogen level is very contributory to atrophic vaginitis with vaginal wall thinning, and the resultant decreased lubrication, dryness, burning, and painful intercourse women can have if estrogen is not replaced. Furthermore, the low estrogen levels also contribute to decreased blood supply to the pelvis and slower nerve transmission, associated with decreased orgasmic potential.

Since all ovarian hormones are decreased in the menopausal patient, so is testosterone, which is classified in a group of hormones known as androgens. These are what give women their libido. Women in their 40s have about one half the testosterone women in their 20s do, and the levels continue to drop after menopause. The ovary becomes the major source of testosterone after menopause. Before the change, however, these women had most of their testosterone produced by a chemical pathway from their adrenal glands, where a hormone called DHEA is manufactured. DHEA-S, or dehydroepiandrosterone sulfate is the major prohormone that is converted to testosterone. This is the pathway that drys up in the post-menopausal patient.

Everyone wants their hormone levels "checked", and if you read any lay woman's magazine, they tell you to ask your doctor to do this.

Simple right? No, it's not, unfortunately. The value of assessing free (not total) testosterone levels is unclear, because available assays are _not_ _reliable_ enough or sensitive enough to measure in women. Over and over, we have discovered libido is not necessarily correlated with free testosterone levels in all women. Testosterone therapy does seem to help libido however in about 50 % of menopausal patients.

Trials have been done that show the menopausal woman gets best relief of her hot flashes over a three month time period with a combination of *low* dose estrogen and testosterone together. In second place was high dose estrogen only, and in third place was high dose estrogen with testosterone. The important thing to remember is that if the estrogen levels are too high, a protein in the blood called SHBG (Sex Hormone Binding Globulin) rises. The levels of this blood protein are always inversely correlated with free testosterone levels. So high estrogen levels lead to higher SHBG levels, and this further lowers free testosterone. It's the free testosterone level that counts!

Studies have also been done that shown that the route of administration of the estrogen is very important. CEE (conjugated conjugated estrogens) increase SHBG around 100%, oral micronized estrogen increases it 45 %, and transdermal estrogen increases it the least 12%. Since a higher increase in SHBG causes a lower free testosterone, the oral CEE will depress free testosterone more than the transdermal (patch) will. So the estrogen in a patch form will result in a higher free testosterone level than an oral product.

Currently, the FDA is looking over the data from a new testosterone patch for women which may well become the first FDA approved product for administration to women. Hopefully this will be a huge breakthrough for menopausal patients!

Currently Available Prescription Testosterone Therapies

It is very important to realize that there are currently <u>no</u> FDA-approved testosterone products for sexual dysfunction in women (just men). Products have to be prescribed *off label* by your provider for this indication.

Testosterone injections often result in *too high* a level of testosterone, but these patients feel exceptionally well initially. The major long term drawbacks are testosterone excess symptoms: growth in facial and body hair, deepening of the voice, oily skin, increased acne, and weight gain, clitoral enlargement, mood swings (especially anger), and adverse cholesterol (lipid) changes. Also, since testosterone is converted to estrogen, one may get excess estrogen effects. On the beneficial side, half the time we obtain a better libido, less depression, and increased muscle tone.

Please note that if androgen levels are kept within physiologic ranges, the negative effects of testosterone therapy are minimal. This is tricky because remember blood testing is unreliable, physiologic response differs, and much of current day clinical monitoring of androgen levels is by subjective evaluation.

Oral

Methytestosterone
Testosterone Undecanoate

Intramuscular Injections

Testosterone Proprionate, Cypionate, or Enantrate

Subcutaneous Pellets

Testosterone Proprionate Pellets

Transdermal

Testosterone Patches, Gel, Emulsion, and Spray
(Please note that current testosterone patches for men should not be used, and are too high for women: Androderm and Testoderm. Also, the gel Androgel has the same problem, and should not be used in women.)

Other Forms

Testosterone Vaginal Rings

Testosterone Sublingual

Combined Oral Estrogen and Testosterone

Estratest (oral esterified estrogen and methyl testosterone) 0.625 mg. EE+ 1.25 mg. MT, and 1.25 mg. EE+ 1.25 mg. MT). Estratest is an exceptionally good product for the menopausal patient in general, and is indicated for those hot flashes unresponsive to estrogens.

Compounded Testosterone Cream or Ointment (2%)

This may be applied to any skin surface, including the inner thigh, vagina, or clitoris. It is well absorbed through the skin, but it is quite easy to have too high a level of absorption, and have just as many side effects as above.

ɕ૩ ɕ૩ ɕ૩

In some women, these testosterone products work incredibly well. There is an increase in sexual desire, frequency of fantasies, and sexual arousal. One of my 76 year old patients after her first low dose testosterone injection within a week was wearing out her husband out so badly that he presented to my office begging me lower her dose even further. She wanted sex three times day, and has often has later joked that she was going to take care of him in the parking lot before driving home! I lowered her next injection dosage......she and he husband are extremely happy, and she has minimal side effects. So one can see that testosterone usage is somewhat tricky. Close subjective followup is necessary by the clinician, as well as following serum lipid levels.

Monitoring blood levels of free testosterone or free androgen index (Total testosterone/ SHBG) for women using topical products is advised as a safety measure. However, commercial laboratory measurements are quite variable. So, in summary, this is tricky in today's environment.

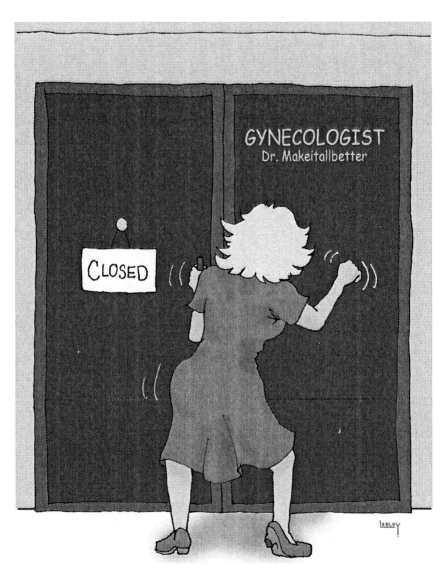

You can't wait to go to your Gyno for your HRT refill!

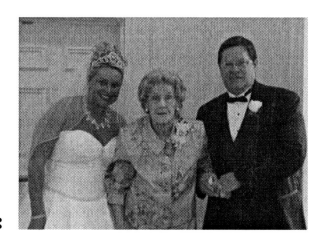

Chapter 6:

The Menopause And Your Bones: An Ounce of Prevention IS Worth a Pound of Cure!

By Neil C. Boland, M.D., F.A.C.O.G.

As menopausal practitioners, we have to be vigilant among our patients as to which of them will eventually develop osteoporosis. For example, my brother and niece in the picture above is holding up my dear mother Louise. She was at one time 5 feet 8 inches tall, and now at age 91 is only 5 feet 1 inch tall, a full 7 inches shorter than she was in the 1950s.

Unfortunately, this problem is a familial one, and alendronate (Fosamax) which my mother is now taking was not FDA-approved until the late 1990's. Had she been able to take that medication several decades ago, she very likely would have been able to stabilize and preserve most of her prior height. She has already had one hip replacement, and struggles with a walker. Our baby boomer generation has an important advantage over our parents--- we can diagnose and treat osteoporosis earlier than my mother could. It's more than just a problem of mobility limitation, joint pain, and surgical hospitalization. At least 20% of patients *die* of complications of a single hip fracture. We are presenting selected excerpts below from the NAMS (North American Menopause Society) 2006 Position Statement on Osteoporosis, as referenced in Recommended Reading.

Osteoporosis is the most common bone disorder affecting humans. It is a skeletal disorder characterized by compromised bone strength predisposing a person to an increased risk of fracture. Bone strength (and, hence, fracture risk) is dependent on both bone quality and bone mineral density (BMD). Expressed as grams of mineral per area or volume, BMD at any given age is a function of peak bone mass (reached around age 30 years) and how much bone is subsequently lost. Other qualities of bone other than BMD are difficult or impossible to measure in clinical practice.

To standardize values from different bone densitometry tests, results are reported as either a Z-score or a T-score, with both expressed as standard deviation (SD) units.

- The T-score is calculated by comparing current BMD to the mean peak BMD of a normal, young adult population of the same gender. For women, the reference database is white (non-race-adjusted) women aged 20 to 29 years. Use of T-scores is the preferred choice for postmenopausal women.

- Z-score is based on the difference between the woman's BMD and the mean BMD of a reference population of the same gender, age, and ethnicity.

The World Health Organization (WHO) definition of osteoporosis in a postmenopausal woman as a BMD T-score less than or equal to -2.5 at the total hip, femoral neck, or lumbar spine (posterior-anterior, not lateral). If anatomic factors such as obesity or arthritis make measurements invalid, the distal one-third radius bone density may be considered a diagnostic site. However, the relationship between the T-score at this site and fracture risk has not been yet examined.

In addition to diagnosis through densitometry, osteoporosis can be diagnosed clinically, regardless of the T-score. Presence of a fragility fracture constitutes the clinical diagnosis of osteoporosis.

Peak bone mass is achieved during a woman's third decade of life. *The process of bone loss begins at that time and accelerates at menopause. By age 80, many women have lost, on average, approximately 30% of their peak bone mass. However, osteoporosis is not always the result of bone loss. A woman who does not achieve an adequate peak bone mass as a young adult may have low bone mineralization without substantial bone loss as she ages.*

Osteoporosis has no warning signs. Often, the first indication of the disease is a fracture. Nearly all nonvertebral fractures are caused by a fall; however, vertebral fractures often occur without a fall. Wrist fracture, which tends to occur at a younger age than vertebral or hip fracture, may also be an early clinical expression of osteoporosis.

Osteoporosis is categorized as either primary or secondary. Primary osteoporosis is usually due to bone loss that occurs with aging. Secondary osteoporosis is a result of medications (eg, glucocorticoids), certain medical conditions (eg, such as multiple myeloma), or diseases (eg, malabsorption) that adversely affect skeletal health.

The primary clinical goal of osteoporosis management is to reduce fracture risk. This may be accomplished by slowing or stopping bone loss, increasing bone mass or improving bone architecture, maintaining or increasing bone strength, and minimizing factors that contribute to falls. Management strategies include general preventive health measures and pharmacologic interventions.

Prevalence

Most cases of osteoporosis occur in postmenopausal women, and the prevalence of the disorder as defined by low BMD increases with age. Data from the Third National Health and Nutrition Examination Survey (NHANES III) indicate that 13% to 18% of white American women aged 50 or older have osteoporosis of the hip, which the survey defined as above.

For an American woman at age 50 years, the risk of suffering an osteoporotic fracture in her remaining lifetime has been estimated at 40%, with two thirds of the fractures occurring after age 75. The estimated remaining lifetime risks after age 50 years for hip, vertebral, and forearm fracture are 17.5%, 15.6%, and 16.0%, respectively.

In the United States, the rates of osteoporosis and fracture vary with ethnicity. In one large study of postmenopausal women from five ethnic groups (white Americans, African Americans, Asian Americans, Hispanic Americans, and Native Americans), African Americans had the highest BMD, while Asian Americans had the lowest; only the BMD differences for African Americans were not explained by differences in weight. After adjusting for weight and BMD, white Americans and Hispanic Americans had the highest risk of osteoporotic fracture, followed by Native Americans, African Americans, and Asian Americans. The age-adjusted lifetime risks of hip fracture in US women are 17% for white Americans, 14% for Hispanic Americans, and 6% for African Americans. These differences, however, may be related more to body size than to race.

Morbidity and Mortality

Hip fractures cause up to a 25% increase in mortality within 1 year of the incident. Approximately 25% of women require long-term care after a hip fracture, and 50% will have some long-term loss of mobility.

Fractures at other sites can also result in serious morbidity. Vertebral fractures occur, on average, in a woman's mid-70s. Multiple or severe vertebral fractures may cause substantial pain as well as loss of height and exaggerated thoracic kyphosis. Spinal pain and deformity can greatly restrict normal movement, including bending and reaching.

Osteoporotic fractures take a psychological toll as well. Hip and vertebral fractures and the resultant pain, loss of mobility, changed body image, and loss of independence can have a significant impact on self-esteem.

How Does This Happen?

Bone remodeling is the process of bone resorption and bone formation. At the cellular level, osteoclasts (the bad cells) promote bone resorption by stimulating the production of acid and enzymes that dissolve bone mineral and proteins. Osteoblasts (the good cells) promote bone formation by creating a protein matrix consisting primarily of collagen, which is soon calcified, resulting in mineralized bone.

In normal bone remodeling, bone resorption is balanced by bone formation. Bone loss occurs when there is an imbalance between bone resorption and bone formation, resulting in a decrease in bone mass and an increase in the risk of fracture.

Menopause is associated with a few years of rapid bone loss attributed to lower circulating levels of estrogens, related primarily to the loss of estrogen-mediated inhibition of bone resorption without a fully compensatory increase in bone mass.

Who Is At Risk For Osteoporosis?

Advanced age

Low BMD

Previous fracture (other than skull, facial bone, ankle, finger, and toe) as an adult

History of hip fracture in a parent

Thinness [body weight <127 lb (57.7 kg) or low BMI (<21 kg/m^2)]

Current smoking, any amount

Low calcium or vitamin D intake

More than two alcoholic drinks per day

Oral or intramuscular glucocorticoid use for >3 mo

Increased fall risk

Impaired vision

Dementia

Poor health/frailty

Low physical activity

History of recent falls

(BMD= bone mineral density; BMI= body mass index).

*Courtesy of North American Menopause Society 2006 Position Statement on Osteoporosis

Treatment-induced changes in BMD do not always correlate well with reductions in vertebral fracture risk. In addition, fracture risk reductions in response to antiresorptive therapy occur much more rapidly than discernible BMD changes. For example, significant fracture risk reduction has been reported after 6 months of risedronate (Actonel) therapy, although minimal BMD increases were observed at that time.

A balanced diet plays an important role in bone development and maintenance of bone health throughout life. Both calcium and vitamin D have well-known roles in bone metabolism. Adequate intake of calcium (1,200 mg. daily) and vitamin D (400 mIU daily) is required throughout life for a woman to achieve her genetically determined peak bone mass and to maintain optimal bone mass and strength after peak bone mass is attained.

Low vitamin D intake has been linked to impaired muscle strength, increased fall risk, and increased fracture risk along with increased rates of bone loss. Furthermore, treatment with vitamin D has been found to reduce fracture risk in elderly postmenopausal women, although not in all studies. Elderly postmenopausal women have an increased risk of hip fracture associated with low dietary calcium intake.

There is general agreement that weight-bearing exercises confer a positive effect on the musculoskeletal system and that weight-bearing exercises (eg, walking, running, step aerobics, gymnastics) provide the greatest osteogenic (bone building) stimulus.

Regular exercise has been associated with reduced fracture risk. Exercise also appears to reduce the risk of falls by increasing muscle mass, strength, and balance, although it is unclear whether exercise affects the risk of fracture from falls that do occur. Long-term immobilization, such as prolonged bed rest, has been associated with rapid and significant bone loss.

What Medical Conditions Can Cause Secondary Osteoporosis?

Medications:

Oral or intramuscular use of glucocorticoids for >3 months

Excessive thyroxine doses

Aromatase inhibitors

Long-term use of certain anticonvulsants (eg, phenytoin)

Heparin

Cytotoxic agents

Gonadotropin-releasing hormone agonists or analogues

Depo-Provera contraceptive Usage (prolonged)

Immunosuppressives (eg, cyclosporine)

Genetic disorders

Hemochromosiderosis

Osteogenesis Imperfecta

Hypophosphasia

Hypercalciuria

Vitamin D deficiency

Endocrinopathies

Cushing's Syndrome

Gonadal insufficiency (primary and secondary)

Hyperthyroidism

Type I Diabetes Mellitus

Primary Hyperparathyroidism

Gastrointestinal Diseases

Chronic liver disease (eg, Primary Biliary Cirrhosis)

Malabsorption syndromes (eg, Celiac Disease, Crohn's Disease)

Total Gastrectomy Surgery

Billroth I Gastroenterostomy

Other disorders and conditions

Multiple Myeloma

Lymphoma and Leukemia

Systemic Mastocytosis

Nutritional Disorders (eg, Anorexia Nervosa)

Rheumatoid Arthritis

Chronic Renal Disease

* Courtesy NAMS 2006 Position Statement on Osteoporosis

All postmenopausal women should be assessed for risk factors associated with osteoporosis and fracture. This assessment requires a history, physical examination, and any necessary diagnostic tests. Blood Testing may or may not have to be performed.

Blood Workup of Osteoporosis

Test	Diagnostic result	Possible secondary cause
Complete blood cell count	Anemia	Multiple myeloma
Serum calcium	Elevated	Hyperparathyroidism
	Low	Vitamin D deficiency, GI malabsorption

Serum 25-hydroxyvitamin D	Low	GI malabsorption, celiac disease
Serum albumin	Used to interpret serum calcium	
Serum alkaline phosphatase	Elevated	Vitamin D deficiency, GI malabsorption, hyperparathyroidism, Paget's disease
Urinary calcium excretion	Elevated	Renal calcium leak, multiple myeloma, metastatic cancer involving bone, hyperparathyroidism, hyperthyroidism
	Low	GI malabsorption, inadequate intake of calcium and vitamin D

*Courtesy NAMS 2006 Position Statement on Osteoporosis

Calcium

Evidence has established the role of adequate calcium intake on bone health, primarily in increasing BMD and improving the efficacy of therapeutic agents. Calcium has not been shown to have a positive effect on fracture risk. However, in the Women's Health Initiative (WHI) trial, hip fractures were significantly reduced in older women who were adherent to the calcium regimen.

Calcium requirements increase with advancing age, particularly after menopause, owing in part to both reduced intestinal calcium absorption and renal calcium conservation. The primary factor influencing the amount of calcium absorbed is the amount of calcium ingested. Here are the most recent NIH/ NAS Recommendations:

National Academy of Sciences Age 31-50	1,000 mg
Age 51 and older	1,200 mg
National Institutes of Health Premenopausal women aged 25-50	1,000 mg
Postmenopausal women younger than age 65 and using estrogen therapy	1,000 mg
Postmenopausal women not using estrogen therapy	1,500 mg
All women aged 65 and older	1,500 mg

Adapted from the National Institutes of Health and the National Academy of Sciences.

Vitamin D

The nutrient vitamin D is essential for the intestinal absorption of calcium. The current National Academy of Sciences recommended dietary intake for vitamin D is 400 IU/day for women aged 51 to 70 years and 600 IU/day for women older than age 70. In addition, NAMS recommends intake of 700 to 800 IU/day for women at risk of deficiency because of inadequate sunlight exposure, such as older, frail, chronically ill, housebound, or institutionalized women or those who live in northern latitudes. Doses as high as 2,000 IU/day are safe. Much higher doses may introduce risks such as hypercalciuria and hypercalcemia.

Who Should Undergo Prescription Therapy for Prevention or Treatment of Osteoporosis?

We would treat with medication any person with osteoporosis, a history of a vertebral fracture, or a BMD of -1.5 or less. Several pharmacologic options are available for osteoporosis therapy, including:

1) Bisphosphonates: alendronate (Fosamax), risidronate (Actonel), Ibandronate (Boniva), etidronate (Didronel). These medications work by inhibiting bone reabsorption of calcium.

2) SERM raloxifene (Evista). This is a Selective Estrogen Receptor Modulator, and also works by inhibiting bone reabsorption.

3) Parathyroid Hormone (Forteo) This medication is injectable and fairly expensive, and works by actually building new bone matrix.

4) Estrogens (see below).

5) Calcitonin (Miacalcin nasal spray). This is also a resorption inhibitor.

According to the NAMS 2006 Technical Bulletin on Osteoporosis, no studies have yet been reported in comparison of these therapies for antifracture efficacy.

Adherence to therapy is relatively poor, but still doable. The most common side effects of bisphosphonate therapy are gastrointestinal upset. Very little of the medication is absorbed in the GI tract, so the medication has to be taken on an empty stomach with a 12 oz. glass of water at least one hour prior to a meal. In studies of 6 months to 1 year, adherence rates for prescription drugs ranged from below 25% to 81%, depending on the type of therapy.

Relative to estrogen therapy, the two largest and best controlled trials support the use of estrogens. In the Postmenopausal Estrogen/Progestin Interventions (PEPI) trial, standard daily doses of 0.625 mg conjugated equine estrogens (CEE), with or without a progestogen (either medroxyprogesterone acetate (MPA) or micronized progesterone) for 3 years significantly increased spinal BMD by 3.5% to 5.0%, with a 1.7% increase in hip BMD. More recently, the WHI, a 5-year randomized controlled trial in postmenopausal women aged 50 to 79 years reported that standard doses of daily EPT (0.625 mg CEE plus 2.5 mg MPA) significantly increased spine and total hip BMD by 4.5% and 3.7%, respectively, relative to placebo.

We monitor BMD by performance of Dexascans every 2 years or so. Don't neglect your bones, or you will slowly turn into dust!

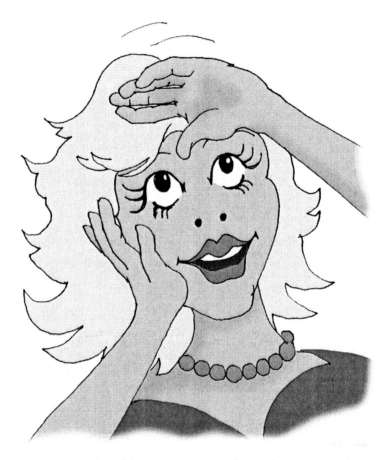

Whenever I feel blue, I just start breathing again!

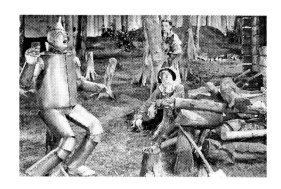

Chapter 7:

The Menopause and Cardiovascular Function:
Making Sense of the WHI Study 2002-2006

By Neil C. Boland, M.D., F.A.C.O.G.

If I Only Had A Heart

Heart and cardiovascular disease is the number one killer of women age 65 or older. Cardiovascular disease is an all inclusive term, which includes atherosclerosis, stroke, coronary vessel disease (angina and heart attack), high blood pressure, congestive heart failure, valvular heart disease, peripheral vascular disease, and cardiac arrhythmias (abnormal heart rhythms). Interactions between these disease processes are complex and beyond the scope of this book. To achieve optimal health in women, it is of paramount importance to exercise on a regular basis, achieve optimal weight, control high blood pressure, monitor cholesterol values, and reduce each individual's risk of abnormal blood clotting.

How Estrogen Helps the Healthy Woman

What role may estrogen play in reduction of cardiovascular risk? Observational studies have shown that estrogen may exert multiple beneficial effects in improving lipid balance, enhancing internal blood vessel lining repair, reducing platelet cohesiveness, and dropping blood pressure. This latter effect is thought to be due to a favorable release of nitric oxide (a vasodilator) from the walls of blood vessels. In addition, estrogen is felt to play a key role in stabilization of plaques in blood vessel walls that can rupture, triggering a blood clot which can cause a heart attack and stroke.

Estrogen's Effects on Cholesterol

Oral estrogens raise HDL (good cholesterol) and lower LDL (bad cholesterol) which is beneficial. However orals raise triglyceride levels, which is potentially adverse. It has been suggested that the single best predictor of cardiovascular risk in women are serum levels of HDL. The higher the HDL, it is felt the lower the cardiovascular risk. The PEPI trial (Postmenopausal Estrogen/ Progestin Interventions) showed that either estrogen alone or combined with progesterone will significantly increase HDL and lower LDL, although slightly less with the addition of a type of progesterone.

Transdermal estrogens (patches) also increase HDL and lower LDL (slightly less than orals), but have no effect on triglycerides, unlike orals. (Patches also do not lower free testosterone as much as orals). It is felt the difference in lipid effects with patches is due to the avoidance of the first pass effect through the liver.

It is well known that estrogen and progesterone hormonal receptors are present in all blood vessel walls, including the coronary arteries, which supply blood to the heart muscle itself. Menopause induces changes in these receptors. In addition, menopause changes coagulation balances, increases insulin resistance, and exaggerates bodily stress responses. It also causes changes in cholesterol balances by increasing LDL (bad cholesterol), total cholesterol, and triglyceride levels. Over time, it also decreases HDL (good cholesterol) as well. None of these normal changes in the aging female are beneficial. The role that estrogen plays in the menopausal vascular theater is complex.

2002 -2004 WHI Findings: Bad For the Unhealthy Woman

We have already gone over the 2002 WHI findings relative to heart attack and stroke risk in Chapter 4 related to combination estrogen and progesterone versus estrogen only. In the WHI population, both disease processes showed a *slightly worse outcome* with both types of therapies. *However, it cannot be emphasized enough that the WHI population studied was much older, more obese, more hypertensive, more diabetic, and had more preexistent inherent cardiovascular risk factors than the younger healthier 45-55 year old who presents to our office daily with severe hot flashes. The two populations are totally different.* On reanalysis of the WHI data in 2006, we are starting to discover the most important information of all!

During the week of March 1, 2004, the National Institutes of Health stopped the estrogen-only phase of the Women's Health Initiative (WHI). The WHI found an increased risk of stroke and no reduction in the risk of heart disease in postmenopausal women who had had a hysterectomy. In February 2004 , the American Heart Association updated its Guidelines for Cardiovascular Disease Prevention in Women with new recommendations for HT. *Combined hormone therapy is not recommended for the prevention of heart disease and stroke in postmenopausal women.* The Guidelines recommended a conservative approach to the use of estrogen-alone hormone therapy until further research is available. In fact, the FDA now requires drug companies to post a "black box warning" that all estrogens with or without progestins should not be used for *secondary* prevention of cardiovascular disease. *This means if a patient already has the disease, we cannot prevent further progression of the disease with hormones.*

2006 WHI Findings: Healthy For The Healthy Woman

It is very important to mention that in 2006, a reanalysis of the original WHI patients was published, and patients were stratified into age groups. This study was published and showed a statistically significant 37% *REDUCTION* in heart attack risk in women in the 50-59 age group (remember this is the younger WHI group!) *So we are now seeing that HT gives different risk profiles contingent upon the age of the patient and her inherent cardiovascular risk profile.*

Conclusions & Case Studies

So what does this all mean to the average postmenopausal woman? Does an average postmenopausal woman even exist? Personally, *I think this evaluation has much less to do with chronologic age, and more to do with the physiologic age of each individual woman.*

We should consider two distinctly different types of patients. For example, consider the 45 year old nearly postmenopausal woman in the workforce who is 5'2" tall and weighs 230 pounds, with a blood pressure of 146/92, a waist measurement of 42 inches, a fasting blood sugar of 115 (high) , a total cholesterol of 256 (high), and HDL of 42 (low), an LDL of 192 (high), and triglycerides are 220. Her father died of an MI at 52. She smokes ¾ packs cigarettes a day, and is "trying to quit", but says she is "all stressed out right now". Her exercise consists of a brisk walk to the refrigerator five times a day. She is very distressed because she has awful hot flashes at 3 AM nightly. Should she be offered hormonal therapy? Absolutely NOT. It is very likely she has at least some significant underlying atherosclerosis. Her cardiovascular risk factors for MI and stroke are high, and relative potential benefits are low.

A second patient (who is real) would be a retired 59 year old woman, 5'7" tall , and weighing 122 pounds. She did not undergo menopause until age 57. She runs 80 miles per week, and looks trim and fit. Her blood pressure is 116/72 (low), resting pulse is 62, fasting blood sugar is 76 (low), total cholesterol is 199, HDL is 130 (high), and LDL is 60 (low), and triglycerides are 87 (low). She has rather thin bone structure because she had to take a long course of steroids for asthma. Her mother had a "hump" in her back in her later years, and had to have a hip replacement. She has no family history of cardiovascular disease or stroke, and she is a never smoker. She too feels terrible because she cannot sleep some nights due to flashes and sweats. Should she be offered hormonal therapy? YES! From a cardiac standpoint, she is low risk. It is her choice to take hormonal therapy or try CAMH medications (see Chapter 9) . She also should have been evaluated many years ago for bone loss with DEXA scanning. If she exhibited a DEXA T-score of -1.5 or lower, I would also offer her bisphosphonate oral therapy to help strengthen her bones, along with estrogen therapy. Benefits are high, and risk is low.

Obviously, most patients do not come into the office with such clear cut risk profiles. But I think consciously or not, clinicians tend to put patients into either low, medium, or high risk cardiovascular profiles. Based on the 2006 WHI findings, we are now confidently able to offer or withhold HT selectively to patients based on our classification of each individual's cardiac risk profile (among multiple other factors).

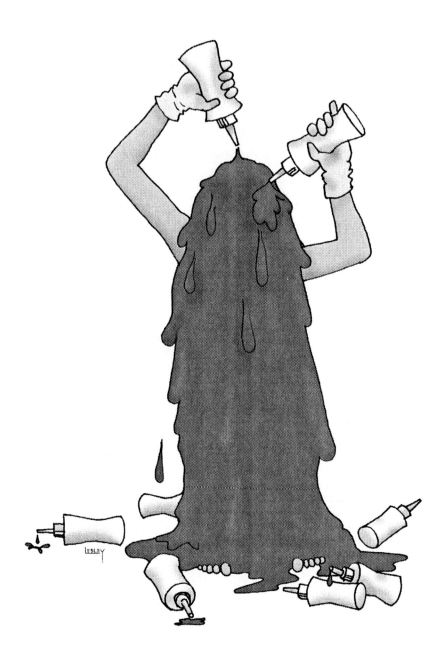

When you start to tint your hair
from your head to your toes!

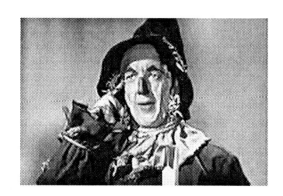

Chapter 8:

Mood Swings And Changes In Cognitive Function: Being Proactive, Not Reactive, Or I Got A New Attitude!

By Neil C. Boland, M.D., F.A.C.O.G.

The Myths

As a long practicing clinician, I have found that two enduring old wives tales or myths seem to come up repetitively about the menopausal woman. Neither myth is true, and they seem to be at opposite ends of the spectrum.

Myth #1: Menopause is filled with several years of distressing mood swings, anxiety, panic attacks, and very serious depression *for all women.* Lots of patients think they will turn into emotional basket cases and need to be institutionalized. Statistics show that women in their forties and fifties are no more likely to become depressed than women of other ages, and are actually less likely than women in their twenties and thirties, who face different forms of stress.

Myth #2: Menopause is *all in your mind*. In 2003, a major East Coast newspaper editorial was written explaining that almost all menopausal symptoms were simply figments of women's imaginations and nothing more than propaganda by pharmaceutical companies who are promoting sales of hormone therapy.

As we have explained in previous chapters, menopause is a natural process most women will have to face at some point in their lives. Its symptoms in most patients are real, and can have profound effects on their skin, brain, bones, teeth, eyes, moods, sleep, and reproductive organs. The menopausal syndrome of estrogen deficiency, as we call it, is no more psychosomatic in origin than diabetes is a psychosomatic deficiency of insulin. Some patients have more severe menopausal symptoms than others, but it's *not in your mind*.

Ever heard your neighbor say she went through menopause, and it was really no big deal? She didn't experience many physiologic or psychological negative changes at all she says? Her irregular periods just stopped, and it somehow never really bothered her? She just shrugs and smiles. I count that individual as fortunate, but she is in a definite *minority.* As physicians, we don't totally understand what makes some patients have minimal, is any symptoms, and others have the full blown syndrome.

Depression in The PM Patient

Most individuals do experience some degree of fatigue, sleep disturbance, memory loss, irritability, and/ or difficulty in concentration. Many women find they can become teary eyed at the drop of a hat from nothing more than a television dishwasher liquid commercial. The fact remains that many women can become somewhat depressed around menopause, and the biochemical origin is still unclear, possibly estrogen deficiency or changes in hormonal levels. As we described in an earlier chapter of this book, low estrogen causes us to have higher levels of the enzyme monoamine oxidase in our brain, which breaks down our four major brain neurotransmitter hormones, which is not a good thing. Other origins of depression point to the psychological effects of stress, sleep deprivation, loss of general health, socioeconomic changes, and even possible loss of self-esteem. Also, certain other disease processes, such as Lyme Disease, CFS (Chronic Fatigue Syndrome), and Epstein-Barr virus can cause depression.

Is It Really PMS Instead?

We addressed PMS, or Pre-menstrual Tension Syndrome, in other areas of this book. We frequently find that many patients develop PMS symptoms (bloatedness, malaise, irritability, hostility, panic attacks, and food cravings) suddenly in their forties and continue it until menopause. However, PMS can be present in women of any active menstrual age. Also there is some overlapping of PMS symptoms with those of the perimenopausal patient. I personally feel they are different diseases, but a really objective diagnostic distinction is neither possible nor actually terribly relevant. PMS patients seem, in general, to respond very well to the SSRI antidepressant class of medications.

Can These Mood Swings Be Treated?

I have found that if menopausal patients require antidepressant medication, it may or may not work unless some from of estrogen is administered first. In some patients, simply the estrogen therapy alone works for the depression without the antidepressant. If I am unsuccessful in managing their depression at follow-up appointments, they are referred for psychiatric consultation, because of the possibility that other mood disturbances may have emerged or become uncovered by menopause.

Does HT (Hormonal Therapy) work in treatment of all these mental changes? Fortunately, yes, and most of the time almost *miraculously!* Patients return to my office usually unable to contain their happiness in discovery it really wasn't "just in their mind". They sleep so much better, and as such, their mental clarity and focus return, as well their former energy level, and their moods stabilize. They throw away their tubes of progesterone creams which never really worked that well anyway (same as placebo), as proven in multiple scientific studies really fail miserably. At this point, we then frequently have to get them off the addictive sleeping pills and tranquilizers they have been getting from their sister-in-law, and have them face the insidious problem of alcoholism they may have developed trying to get a good night's sleep.

We usually spend a great deal of time reassuring patients about risks, e.g., the miniscule, if any, increase (0.8%) in breast cancer risk they may encounter if they have to take combination estrogen and progesterone products, if the WHI study is even applicable to younger patients (age 50-59, which it probably is not). We discuss the increase in thrombotic stroke risk and thromophlebitis with estrogen products (about 3%). We discuss that HT may cause a slight increase in heart attack risk in the older patient (also a tiny fraction of one percent). The critical question we now ask them: Since this is your own heathcare decision, are these risks acceptable to you, not for a lifelong commitment, but for a limited time period of your life as you transition into a symptom free post-menopausal patient?

We then discuss the positive benefits of HT: reduced risks of breast cancer if they are taking an estrogen only product, reduced colon cancer risk, reduced uterine cancer risk (if taking combined therapy), reduction in heart attack risk (37% drop) found in patients between age 50-59 without cardiovascular risk factors, reduced risk of osteoporosis, reduced dental and eye problems, better moods, better sleep, better memory, better overall cognitive function, significantly improved ability to have marital relations, better skin, and less wrinkles. It ALWAYS comes up whether or not hormones make one gain weight….NO, not so, according to multiple studies. (In fact, patients on HT of any type weigh slightly less than women not taking HT.)

I always advise these patients to increase exercise, enlarge their social support networks, make new friends, reestablish old family ties if possible, or take up a new hobby, such as yoga, Pilates, meditation, or swimming. Also, I emphasize it is often important for these patients to reinvigorate their spousal or significant other relationships in their lives. Above all, stay mentally active……..read, read, read, do crossword puzzles, learn a new skill by taking a new college course, learn a new language, take up a new musical instrument, or volunteer your mental skills for teaching or serving the less fortunate of society. The mind is just like other organ we possess………use it or lose it.

I cannot overemphasize the problem of sleep deprivation some menopausal women experience, and how it negatively impacts this stage of their lives. It is known that the estrogen deficiency of the menopausal or perimenopausal woman causes vasomotor symptoms, which include hot flashes. The flashes cause these patients to have less REM sleep, which is where the process of dreaming occurs. This is the stage of the sleep cycle we all need in order to feel refreshed and rejuvenated when we awaken. So these patients emerge from bed feeling less than their best. Sleeplessness causes us to feel mentally defocused, irritable, fatigued, depressed, and loose our sense of well-being. So, if you are dreaming during your sleep, count that as a beneficial sign!

Could I have Alzheimer's Syndrome?

Most of us will live long enough either to witness the steady transformation of a loved family member or friend from a healthy active productive member of society to an individual impaired by significant declines in cognitive function. Alzheimer's Syndrome (AD) is a progressive dementing disorder that impairs thinking, memory, and behavior. This disease affects more than 4.5 million Americans, and claims more than 100,000 of them annually. The prevalence of AD doubles every five years after age 65, and affects about half of all individuals age 85 and older. It can occur in middle age, and memory loss is the first sign of this disorder. The memory loss is that of recent memory, that is, what occurred in the past few minutes. These individuals however, can usually recall distant past events in great detail.

These patients can have word finding difficulties, a tendency to get lost, time and place disorientation, and complex task performance impairment (like addressing and mailing a letter). Eventually, the patient may even be unable to bathe or dress themselves, and then loose the ability to communicate with even family members.

Women in their forties and fifties, not surprisingly, become quite concerned when they have difficulties remembering names, appointment times, and where they left their keys. Indeed this has spurred the development of an entire industry of over the counter memory remedies, vitamins, herbs, and other memory aids. Is this a manifestation of declining estrogen levels, or Alzheimer's Syndrome?

Dose of Reality Testing from WHIMS

Currently, we really aren't certain of the role estrogen may or may not play in cognitive function. Initially, earlier studies done in Utah showed that estrogen may play a role in preventative decline as we age, and gave us a feeling of cautious optimism. The WHIMS study seemed to change our optimistic feelings into a more cautious stance.

The Women's Health Initiative Memory Study (also known as WHIMS) has been finished, relative to the use of estrogen and progestin and to estrogen only. This was a study of over 4,500 participants for four years in patients ages 65-79, evaluated relative to their cognitive function, mild cognitive decline, and dementia. The findings were that estrogen and progestin *do not* protect women from mild cognitive declines, compared with placebo. In addition, the medication shows a very tiny increase in the chance of more severe dementia, but only for women age 65 and over.

This translates into only 23 out of every 10,000 patients for the combined medication and 28 out of every 10,000 patients for estrogen only. This meant an increased risk of 0.0023%, and 0.0028% respectively for the two groups, which is very tiny indeed. Further follow-up is being performed on these patients to determine if cognitive impairment continues after the medication has been terminated.

Please note the WHIMS limited their conclusions only to older women (over age 65), and do not necessarily apply to those women in the 45-55 range just reaching menopause, presumably with less or no atherosclerosis. It is in this younger group of patients that hormonal therapy still holds promise of prevention of cognitive decline and AD, but it must be taken for a much longer time period than four years. Further studies are needed.

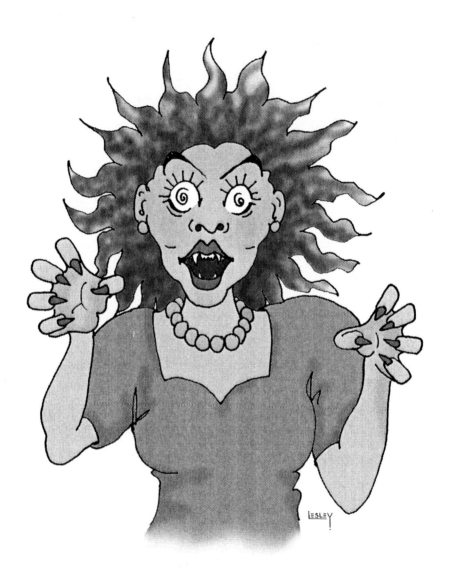

When PMS is a mild thing compared to Menopause!

Chapter 9:

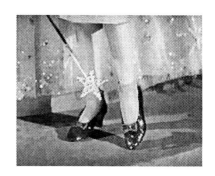

Complementary, Alternative, and Homeopathic Medication(CAHM): Does This Stuff Really Work for Hot Flashes?

By Neil C. Boland, M.D., F.A.C.O.G.

At least 75% of all post-menopausal women suffer from hot flashes of varying severity at some point in their lives. What about those women with severe flashes in whom hormonal therapy is neither medically advisable or declined by the patient? See our list of contraindications to HT (listed in Chapter 3). For these women, the following information is very important.

New Uses for Precription Non-Hormonal Medications

Before I begin this chapter on CAHM, I want to share with you some exciting recent news about several *prescription non-hormonal medications* which work well for treatment of hot flashes. We have known about these for several years, and have been waiting for published scientific data of effectiveness, which has just been done.

Gabapentin (Neurontin)

An article published July, 2006 in the green journal (Obstetrics and Gynecology, July 2006; No. 1: 41-48) showed that the medication *gabapentin* (trade name Neurontin) works *equally as well as estrogen* for reduction in number and severity of flashes. This medication was approved by the FDA in 1994 for seizure control. It can be prescribed off label in doses of 400 mg capsules beginning once at night. Then gradually the dosage can be titrated (increased) up daily over the next 12 days to two capsules three times a day (2,400 mg). Its potential major side effects can be headache, dizziness, and disorientation in some patients. Please keep in mind all medications have potential side effects, and just because it is listed does not mean you personally will experience them, especially if you ease into the recommended doses gradually. As a clinician, what I like about gabapentin is its excellent safety profile and compatibility with other medications.

I recall one particular patient about two years ago who presented to me as a new patient. She was 52 and menopausal, with no period in over a year, and had not slept at all "for over a year". Her hot flashes were so severe she emanated heat from inches away. She could barely walk, hold her eyes open, or speak in coherent sentences. She was severely nicotine addicted, along with almost all the other usual complaints of menopause. She was totally refractory to all types of estrogen therapies, testosterone, and all the usual over the counter remedies. Nothing seemed to work.

Then I started her on gabapentin, gradually increasing her dose to 2,400 mg. per day, seeing her on a weekly basis. The gradual positive transformation was the most remarkable one I have ever seen. Her hot flashes stopped and she began sleeping. She regained her usual cognitive function, and could now balance her checkbook. Her depressed mood disappeared. She stopped smoking and began to exercise. Two months later, she even looked completely differently. Her husband was astounded and delighted, and she is still on gabapentin today.

Venlafaxine (Effexor)

This is an antidepressant which works via the serotonin and norepinephrine pathways. We don't completely understand the exact mechanism by which it works for hot flashes, but placebo controlled studies show that it is at least 61% effective compared to controls in hot flash reduction at the dose of 75 mg XR. Again, this is off label. I start them on 37.5 mg. daily for 7 days, then increase the dose to 75 mg. thereafter. Doses above 75 mg. daily show no increase in efficacy. I have had many breast cancer patients try this regimen with excellent results. Side effects are dry mouth, dizziness, appetite suppression, nausea, and constipation. I have found other antidepressants, such as fluoxitine (Prozac) and paroxetine (Paxil) to be less effective for hot flash management.

Clonidine (Catapres)

This is an antihypertensive medication that is sometimes used for mild hot flashes, but it is less effective than gabapentin and the newer antidepressants. It is used in an oral dose of 0.05 mg twice daily, but some women may require at least 0.1 mg. twice daily. The clonidine patch, delivering 0.1 mg. daily may also be considered. The main side effects which limit its use are sedation, dry mouth, constipation, and dizziness. Also, it is necessary to taper the dosage from the higher dosages to avoid side effects such as nervousness, agitation, and a rise in blood pressure.

Compounded Bioidentical Hormones

Do not be misled! Forget it. Both the North American Menopause Society and the American College of Ob/ Gyn have published Consensus and/or Committee Opinions that these are potentially dangerous. These are compounded hormones prepared by a pharmacist, and have *not* undergone rigorous scientific clinical testing for safety or effectiveness, unlike prescription hormones. There are also significant issues with purity, potency, and safety, which have to do with the intrinsic risks of compounding these bioidenticals. Again, there is no true scientific evidence to support claims of safety or effectiveness for these hormones. We should all remember that when our post-menopausal patients use prepartions that lack this safety and efficacy data, they are in essence, experimenting with their own bodies. It is their right to do so. It is our responsibility to warn them to do so at their own risk.

These hormonal products can come in many forms, such as creams, orals, injectables, pellet implants, and inhalational hormones. It is remarkable that 34% of these medications fail one or more standard quality tests performed. A full 90% of them fail assay potency testing. Also, purchases of these medications are not typically reimbursed or covered under typical insurance plans.

Salivary Testing

Forget it, because you are wasting your money. There is no scientific evidence at all that hormone levels in saliva are biologically meaningful. Two basic problems exist as saliva is an ultrafiltrate of the blood : 1) there is no correlation between saliva and blood hormonal concentrations that are meaningful, and 2) within the same patient, salivary hormone levels are tremendously variable, depending on diet and time of day. You are simply donating money to charity when you have these done...... usually the charity is the bank account of the laboratory, website, or even "healthcare entity" who orders or processes it for you.

Progesterone Creams

Remember these non-prescription creams have been shown to fail in effectiveness compared to placebo in several prospective randomized studies. Remember that rubbing toothpaste on your skin will work about 20% of the time too because of the placebo effect (please do not do this!). These creams are usually well absorbed across the skin, but we really do not know 1) how much drug you are receiving, 2) safety data, or 3) its true effectiveness.

Phytoestrogens

These are nonsteroidal estrogens with estrogenic activity, usually plant derived. They can be made from over 300 plants, usually legumes, and fall into three categories: isoflavones (found in chickpeas and soybeans) , coumestans, and lignans (found in flaxseeds, whole grains, and selected fruits and vegetables). Isoflavones are the most common type of phytoestrogen, present in soy products, have both estrogenic and antiestrogenic properties, depending on the type of body tissue involved. A phytoestrogen rich diet has been proposed to be a contributing factor in the relatively low incidence of breast cancer and heart disease present in Asian women.

Depending on which of the multiple studies we have reviewed, these phytoestogens have been shown to be approximately 0- 45 % effective in hot flash reduction.

Black Cohosh (Remifemin)

A recent randomized, double blind, multi-center study showed that this herb is effective in hot flash relief, especially in newly menopausal women. It has been extensively used in Europe. NAMS supports the short term use of cohosh because it seems to have a low risk of side effects when used for time periods up to six months. Effects of longer term use are unknown.

Red Clover, Dong Quai, Licorice, Chasteberry, Evening Primrose Oil, and Vitamin E:

Multiple studies have shown these six products are ineffective for flash relief.

<u>Important Beneficial Biologic Effects of Alternative Therapies</u>

1) Soy protein has been shown to reduce total cholesterol and LDL-cholesterol (the bad type), but it has no effect on HDL-cholesterol (the good type). The FDA in 1999 authorized soy manufacturers to say that soy protein reduced the risk of cardiovascular disease.

2) As synthetic isoflavone, called ipriflavone, has been shown to prevent bone loss but not as great as estrogen or alendronate.

3) Soy protein has been associated with some improvement memory and attention span in post-menopausal women.

4) It is felt that phytoestrogens do provide some protective influence against the development of breast cancer.

Conclusions

The entire field of alternative therapies is fascinating. However, serious research in this field to date is sparse, especially as to how these medications compare with hormonal therapy.

Be sure to consult your healthcare professional before taking any herbal treatments or dietary supplements for symptoms of menopause. Herbal products can interfere or interact with other medications you are taking. See the end of Chapter 13 for a complete listing of vitamins, minerals, alternatives, complimentary, and homeopathic medications. Remember that even though the Food and Drug Administration does not give its approval for using medications, that does not mean that you cannot use them on your own or a physician cannot prescribe them off label. However, we clinicians have a duty to inform our patients that there are serious drawbacks to using untested preparations. Hormonal therapy remains the gold standard for hot flash therapy. Anything else must be subjected to the same standard of scientific scrutiny for safety and effectiveness. The patient deserves nothing less.

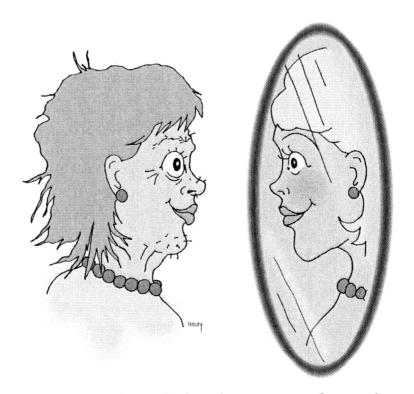

When you can't see the long hairs on your face or chin,
and you think you look just great!

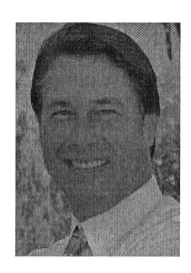

Chapter 10:

Tailoring Hormonal Therapy To The Individual Patient: Frequently Asked Questions of The Gynecologist

By Neil C. Boland, M.D., F.A.C.O.G.

1) Doctor Boland, I am taking estrogen therapy. Does it increase my risk of breast cancer?

Breast cancer is a primary concern and consideration for almost all menopausal women because its incidence increases with age. A woman's random risk of getting it is about a 1 in 8 lifetime chance whether she takes hormones or not.

Keep in mind the WHI study population was older (median age 63), sicker, and more obese than the average of patients who present to the office for hot flash relief (typically age 45-55). It is well known that obesity is a risk factor for breast cancer.

However, even if we look at this older population's 2002 WHI data (utilizing the only type of estrogen and progestin studied), there is only a miniscule increase in cancer risk over controls of 0.8 %, which is tiny (8 tenths of one percent). For estrogen only users, there was a 23% REDUCTION in breast cancer risk compared to controls after a seven year follow up. All this is excellent news! In addition, in 2006, breast cancer is 97-98% curable, with an excellent prognosis in most women. This of course assumes that the patient is doing monthly self breast exams and getting annual mammograms, along with careful annual physical exam by a trained clinician. So, as the WHI study has shown us, the ancient notion that estrogen alone increases breast cancer risk by itself is totally wrong, and can no longer be accepted.

If fear of breast cancer is the only reason a patient is not taking HT, that patient needs to ask herself one fundamental question. Is it worth that tiny increase of 0.8% in risk (or actual DECREASE in risk) for a significant improvement in quality of life? It cannot be generalized for all patients, but the answer for many women after careful consideration is YES. A minority will say no. Again, it is not meant to be a lifetime commitment. The drug literature, which is conservative in approach as mandated by the FDA, says lowest dose effective, for shortest duration of time. I tell those patients about every two years to try to taper or discontinue her HT in order to see if she really needs it for quality of life. I agree with this attempt to get off it eventually not so much from fear of breast cancer, but more from a fear of increased risk of thrombophlebitis and other blood clotting problems (increased risk on HT to about 3%).

Breast cancer is primarily environmental, and not genetic in origin. At least 80% of women diagnosed with breast cancer have no family history whatsoever of it, so I try to dispel the myth of absence of family history as being a protective factor in counseling patients.

I also try to educate patients that we do not feel that it is estrogen that causes or initiates breast cancer. The time course of development of this malignancy is very long indeed. From the first single cancer cell until it is large enough to see on a mammogram (1 mm) is approximately 6.8 years.

It then takes an average of another 3 years (9.8 years total) before it is large enough to palpate on a breast exam as a dominant mass (1 cm., or less than half an inch in diameter). (Remember that even if the mammogram is negative and her confirmatory breast ultrasound shows nothing, that patient always needs a breast biopsy if there is a palpable dominant mass that cannot be otherwise explained.)

A presently evolving school of thought is that women taking combined estrogen and progesterone therapy actually have an <u>earlier</u> diagnosis of breast cancer, if they are in the 1 in 8 patient group who get it. Since it takes about 6.8 years to develop from a single cell to being mammographically detectable, the WHI breast cancers found were already present at the beginning of the study, which lasted only 5.2 years in the combined therapy group . <u>It is felt that not taking hormones does not prevent breast cancer, it just delays the diagnosis</u>. Earlier diagnosis of breast cancer is made, but not more cases of breast cancer. Metaanalyses (large aggregated studies) of breast cancer death rates show that in both E only or E+P hormonal therapy patients who get breast cancer have a more favorable prognosis than patients not taking it because it is detected earlier. These earlier tumors had smaller size and lower grade features (more favorable prognosis). However, the WHI study data contradicted this finding showed slightly larger tumors with 10% more positive nodes in combined E +P users compared to placebo. Again, remember this is not the group of patients who present to the office with hot flashes.

2)   Doctor, what type of medical evaluation is necessary before you feel you can prescribe medication or make a recommendation for treatment of my menopausal symptoms?

First of all, we perform a full history, physical examination, laboratory work, and appropriate imaging studies on the individual menopausal patient. All of this is mandatory and vitally important before decision-

making can occur such that hidden disease processes do not remain undiagnosed and unevaluated.

For example, a careful breast examination may reveal a subtle but worrisome breast mass, which would require diagnostic mammography on an expeditious basis to rule out breast cancer. An enlarged thyroid gland may tip us off that the patient may need further blood testing or scanning. A bone density, for example, may reveal severe osteoporosis, and the patient may require additional medication beyond that of hormonal therapy. An abnormal pelvic exam or suspicious constellation of symptoms may justify the performance of a gynecologic pelvic ultrasound, which may suggest ovarian malignancy. Diagnoses are made. Then, diagnostic blood are imaging studies are performed. Appropriate consultations are ordered, and medical counseling is either done or scheduled.

All of this evaluation is part of what's known as the annual well woman exam (WWE). This includes an initial or interval health history, physical exam, including breast and pelvic exams, with Pap smear if indicated. This includes weight, height, and blood pressure screenings. The baseline mammogram should be done at age 35 or so, and repeated annually starting at age 40. Since breast cancer increases in frequency as women grow older, mammography becomes more important, not less, with each advance in chronologic age. It is a complete myth that after certain age, pelvic exams or mammography is no longer indicated. Remember, most cancers become more common as we age.

Bone density evaluations, also called DEXA scans, are indicated around the time of menopause, and every two years thereafter. If a patient has risk factors for osteoporosis, the DEXA scan needs to be ordered much earlier (see Chapter 6). Colorectal malignancy screening needs to be performed at age 50, and approximately every 5-8 years thereafter. It needs to be performed earlier in patients with a first-degree relative with colorectal cancer or a family history of colon polyps. Pap smears are performed on a regimen recommended by each individual physician, contingent upon individual risk factors for cervical cancer.

In addition, screening for depression, sexual problems, domestic abuse, weight management, and substance addiction should also be performed. In short, we physicians should make every effort to evaluate, manage, triage, and follow medical problems.

3) Are there any health reasons under which you would either never prescribe hormonal therapy (HT) or either be very cautious in doing so? (Contraindications or relative contraindications?)

Yes, absolutely. Absolute or relative contraindications for HT include either active or history of deep venous thrombosis, pulmonary embolus, recent heart attack, severe angina, known peripheral vascular disease, history of stroke or cerebrovascular attack (CVA), untreated hypertension, present anticoagulation therapy, prolonged immobilization, recent surgery requiring immobilization, liver dysfunction, hepatic adenomas, pregnancy, undiagnosed vaginal bleeding, some types of migraine headaches, history of ischemic colitis, most advanced diabetic conditions, advanced or familial dyslipidemias, and most estrogen dependent neoplasia, such as Stage II or higher breast cancer, or Stage II or higher endometrial cancer.

4) Do you ever use birth control pills for treatment of vasomotor symptoms in younger women experiencing vasomotor symptoms? If so, do the same precautions you listed above also apply to birth-control pills for younger women?

Yes, birth control pills (OCPs) are frequently the medication of choice for the perimenopausal patient experiencing heavy or prolonged menses of dysfunctional origin (bleeding not caused by tumor, infection, or pregnancy). OCPs are strong enough to control the bleeding and address the hot flashes quite easily. All of the above contraindications listed above apply also to birth-control pills. One additional contraindication would be any tobacco smoker over age 35. This is because the vasoconstrictive effect of nicotine, combined with the thrombogenic potential of estrogen in OCPs make it a particularly dangerous combination in generation of stroke or CVA. Therefore, all my patients, age 35 or older, have to stop smoking to receive a prescription for OCPs. I will prescribe OCPs up to age 55, and even slightly higher, provided I feel that is medically justified, and no other viable options are available or effective for the patient's vasomotor symptoms.

5) You mentioned that you would prescribe HT to certain categories of patients with either breast or endometrial cancers. Is this true?

Certainly this is permissible under very rare circumstances, and only with a special written informed consent, which I strongly recommend in my office. I've done this no more than 15 times in the last 25 years. Prescribing low dose HT in either Stage I breast or endometrial cancers is off label, meaning that usage of the medication is not FDA approved. This practice is used as well in tertiary care oncology referral centers by highly trained specialists.

These patients have actually been shown to have lower rates of tumor recurrence as well as longer life expectancies compared to controls and a much higher quality of life. The patient selected in this category should have no more than a Stage I cancer, with multiple prospective tumor markers of favorable prognosis, and have absolutely debilitating hot flashes, for which all other therapeutic options have failed. Furthermore, the patient should be required to be totally compliant with monthly self breast examinations, annual mammograms, and pelvic exams. So far, I've had no problems with this approach in my practice, and have very grateful patients.

6) What do you consider valid reasons were prescribing hormonal replacement therapy?

These symptoms may include painful intercourse from the vagina that is not estrogenized or other symptoms of vulvo-vaginal atrophy (which may include vaginal itching and burning, reduction in that lubrication, burning after urination, and even light bleeding after intercourse).

A second category of patient is that of a woman either approaching menopause with irregular periods or has not had a period for at least several months. Most of these are patients that present for evaluation for at least six months from their last menstrual period, and some of them are several years postmenopausal. They complain of severe hot flashes, night sweats, dry skin, irritability, lapses of memory, difficulty concentrating, fuzzy thinking, heart flutters, and insomnia. They frequently stand in front of air conditioner vents, fans, or an open refrigerator door. They complain of sweating multiple times a day, and are generally quite miserable women from these vasomotor symptoms. Generally, the initiation of hormonal therapy in these patients produces within several weeks a brand new woman, and they are among the happiest patients one will find.

A third category patient is that of the immediately post-surgical patient who has undergone removal of her ovaries. These patients experience moderate to severe vasomotor symptoms almost twice as often as a second category. Over 50% of gynecologic surgeons begin HT in the hospital immediately after surgery.

A fourth category of patient would be that of a high risk osteoporosis patient for whom non- estrogen therapies have been considered beforehand. There is definitive evidence from the North American Menopause Society that conjugated equine estrogens (CEE) with the medroxyprogesterone acetate (MPA) reduces potential risk of postmenopausal osteoporosis bone fracture.

Let me say again that I feel our job as a Menopausal Specialist is to outline all potential options available to that patient with treatment of her symptoms. The patient has the right to choose which route she wishes to go. She may choose conventional hormonal therapy, complementary alternative or homeopathic therapy (CAHM), meditation and yoga, or simply do nothing. There are several other prescription non-hormonal medications, which can be utilized with some degree of modest success but with usually other side effects. (See Chapter 9.)

7) How do you as a Menopausal Specialist decide which hormonal replacement product to prescribe for each symptomatic menopausal patient who chooses to initiate HT?

For those patients who still possess a uterus, they will require some form of progestin or progesterone therapy, along with their estrogen component. The current majority opinion in the U.S. is that the function of the progesterone is to provide antagonism to the estrogen component in order to prevent endometrial malignancy and to prevent breakthrough spotting. If the patient does not possess a uterus, she does not need the progesterone. Some very few would argue this point. Combination HT can be administered either in the form of oral pills, which can be either continuous or cyclic, or transdermal patches, which are continuous and kept on the skin of the lower stomach or buttocks at all times, even when bathing.

The progesterone component can be either in oral pills, combined with estrogen in a transdermal patch, or administered in an IUD in the postmenopausal patient. This latter method has been particularly well tolerated by most patients.

If she is already had a hysterectomy, and desires hormonal therapy, she is usually given just plain estrogen. Estrogen can be administered in multiple forms, including oral pills, transdermal patches, injections, vaginal and skin creams, vaginal rings, vaginal pills, and even implantable subcutaneous pellets. Each has advantages and disadvantages, and not all modalities can be tolerated by every patient.

Advantages of hormonal pills include patient convenience, elevation of blood HDL levels, and relatively low cost, compared with transdermal patches. Disadvantages of some pills include possible daily fluctuation in hormonal levels due to metabolism and absorption issues in the gastrointestinal tract and liver.

Advantages of transdermal patches include patient convenience, and they can be used in lower dosages, because they are not dependent on gastrointestinal absorption or subjected to first pass liver metabolism. Patches also have a theoretical advantage of delivering a more consistent blood level of estrogen as well, which may result in fewer headaches and do not raise triglyceride levels the way that oral estrogens do. It has also been speculated that patches may have less effect on gallbladder disease, and do not raise coagulation factors. This may be safer for these patients, including immediate postoperative patients. Disadvantages of patches include higher cost, practical and allergic adhesive issues, and a failure to elevate the more favorable HDL cholesterol component.

I feel is very important that the clinician discuss potential side effects that HT may generate. Generally, patients will have some degree of mastodynia (painful breasts) for the first three or four weeks, which should rapidly go away after that. Most patients who initiate HT will have some degree of spotting for the first 3-6 months and then over the first year gradually disappear. I have found this to be less and less a clinical problem the more highly informed the patient is, and less a problem than it initially seems.

It is highly recommended that only by the drug prescription literature, but also about the WHI studies, that HT be initiated in the lowest possible dose, and administered for the shortest duration of time for alleviation of the patient's symptoms. For some women, that might be one year or less, but it may be as long as 5-10 years or 20 or more. I have some patients in their 80s who refuse to give it up. They go off and hot flashes make their lives miserable. In fact, some of the happiest and healthiest women I have in my practice continue to take hormones into their later years.

8) What do you tell patients who are on HT about a trial of stopping it?

The first thing I tell them is that HT is not meant to be a lifelong commitment because of potential theoretical other risks, cost, and adverse risk/ benefit analysis in some patients. As they age, patients develop other disease processes and are placed on other medications besides HT, which may interact with it. Despite HT being the most intensively studied medication ever studied by mankind, I feel we are just beginning to unlock the mysteries of the profound and significant multi-system aspects of HT…..the good and the bad.

For example, the recent four year Estrogen/ Progestin Replacement Study data (HERS) showed patients had a 35% lower incidence of development of diabetes in patients taking either plain estrogen or combination E+P therapy compared with controls. Even the WHI long term follow up data showed a diabetes development of 3.5% in HT patients versus 4.2% in the placebo group. This suggests that the estrogen deficiency of menopause may be a fundamental element in the development of diabetes. Can you imagine the human morbidity we could prevent in delaying or preventing diabetes in women? We simply need more research, and it is indeed ongoing.

Relative to stopping their estrogen, they can taper off the medication if they like over a period of time, but I have never seen this actually detailed out in a credible scientific publication. I have had the most success just asking patients to stop it cold turkey for 3-4 weeks, starting at age 55 or so (earlier if they like), and repeat this attempt every two- three years. If they can't tell much difference off HT with their quality of life, they can just stop it. However, we should discuss how they feel at their annual checkups.

Some of them who feel they have to have estrogen for quality of life and are taking oral estrogens should be switched to transdermal products if they develop metabolic syndrome, for example.

9) Could you go over which HT products are available today by prescription as low dose oral contraceptive pills? What are their pros and cons?

We tend to prescribe low dose oral contraceptive pills (OCPs) in the perimenopausal patient. Everyone seems to forget that low dose oral contraceptive pills in the 20-35 microgram estradiol range provide excellent bleeding control, contraception, and outstanding control of early menopausal symptoms. This is only true, of course, in the woman who is a non-smoker, and has no other reason for bleeding other than hormonal irregularities. See Chapter 5. All of the same contraindications to HT we have discussed previously apply to OCPs. Smokers over age 35 should not utilize OCPs due to increased risk of stroke and other cardiovascular events. Other contraindications include hypertension, diabetes, history of migraine headaches, or histoies of coronary artery disease, cerebrovascular disease, or venous thromboembolism.

Advantages of birth control pills include suppression of hot flashes, reduced bleeding, reduced menstrual pain, restoration of regular menses, enhanced bone mineral density, decreased surgery for benign ovarian tumors, and reduced breast biopsies for breast disease. Many patients are surprised, and even shocked that OCPs do not increase their risk of breast cancer, but significantly reduce, and in most cases, prevent endometrial and ovarian malignancies. It has been estimated that patients who take birth control pills for 10 years or more have an approximate 50% lifetime reduction in ovarian cancer (same with a tubal sterilization!).

Another available option is that of low dose progestin pills, also known as the mini-pill. However, women taking the mini-pill can experience not only irregular menstrual bleeding but also complete absence of periods altogether. A third option would be that of a progestin-releasing IUD (intrauterine device), which exerts its effects locally. For example, an IUD called Mirena releases a small amount of levonorgestrel (20 micrograms daily). Some patients who who cannot tolerate oral progestins because of side effects seem to do exceptionally well with the IUD in its delivery of progestin to accompany either oral or transdermal estrogen delivery systems. Please remember that some form of progestin should be administered to all patients taking estrogen who have a uterus. Otherwise, those patients are at increased risk for endometrial malignancy. A fourth option would be our old standby Depo-Provera which is an injectable contraceptive for women in any age. However, I do not use it preferentially in the perimenopausal patient because there are so many other options which are safer.

10) What do you do if a patient reports she is taking her medication as usual, but is no longer getting relief of her vasomotor hot flashes from her hormonal therapy?

This is a much more challenging and common problem than one would think in our population, which in South Florida is admittedly somewhat older than most other homogenous menopausal populations in the U. S. in general. The origins of this problem can be: 1) inadequate or decreased absorption of oral hormonal medications (either trade or generic), 2) increased catabolic (breakdown) of the more biologically active estrogens taken systemically by either increased or altered hepatic (liver) function, 3) presence of other medications which may either interfere with either this absorption or catabolism, 4) presence of other substances in the body which alters estrogen's half-life, such as nicotine, which makes estrogen biologically inactive faster by conversion to an inactive estrogen called catecholestrogens, 5) poor dermal adhesiveness of some generic skin patches, and 6) administration of estrogen outside its therapeutic range for that specific individual (keep in mind that serum estrogen levels do not necessarily correlate with how an individual feels). This last point means that if the estrogen level is either too high or too low for that individual, she may not feel vasomotor relief.

I will sometimes check a serum 17-beta-estradiol level in these problem patients to monitor absorption of estrogen, but keep in mind this level can be done meaningfully only in those patients taking only pure 17-beta-estradiol. So, for example, we cannot check a conjugated equine estrogen (Premarin or Prempro) or synthetic conjugated estrogen (Cenestin) level because these mixtures are sometimes 19 or more estrogens . Each of these estrogen types in each pill can have varying degrees of biologic potency. So this is somewhat complex. I've found that simply changing the dose or route of administration, with a tendency to go lower frequently works for us.

11) Doctor, what would you recommend as additional informational resources for the menopausal woman?

I highly recommend <u>www.knowmenopause.com</u>. This is an outstanding source of information for the patient interested in her own participation in medical decision making. It is an informative blend of user-friendly tools and web videos featuring real women who share stories. Real health care professionals also offer advice and guidance for questions and concerns women have at menopause. This is supported by Wyeth Pharmaceuticals. For additional resources, see Resources section at the end of this book.

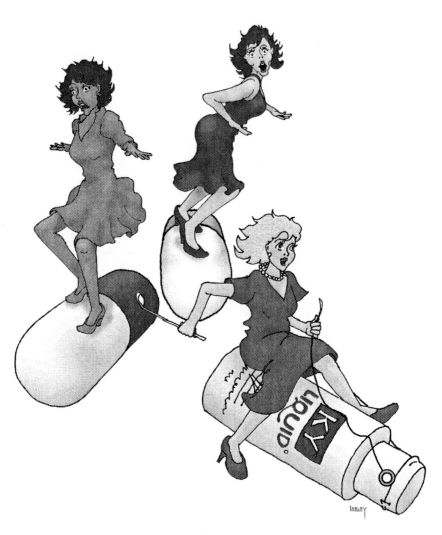

You go to the Pharmacy just to get
KY Liquid and sleeping pills

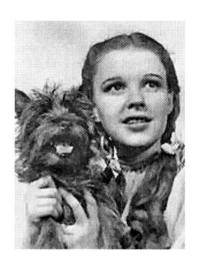

Chapter 11

What to look for in Menopausal skin: Let's stay healthy and happy!

By Linda LaVelle A.T.I.E. I.T.E.C.

Look vibrant, stay healthy, and be happy! These are my goals that my clients have when they come to see me. As a Board Certified Esthetician for over 30 years, my approach with clients has always been varied and different with each skin that I look at. I know that the results of aging skin have equally as much to do with a good skin care regimen and proper nutritional intake, as it has with ones emotional being. My approach to this is the same. I treat the whole of the person rather than just the skin. I want to find out how they work, how their family life is, the stress that they endure, the amount of sports that they involved in, and how much they are on the phone, as well as their hormonal conditions as well as life's ups and downs. So by treating the whole person and I am accomplishing the "Whole Person" rather than just their skin.

You see, traditional skin care programs have failed to prove lasting results. They merely camouflage the visible signs of aging without actually improving the quality and health of the skin.

The program outlined in this chapter is easy to follow and use, unlike any other anti-age book, it is scientifically proven not only to reduce your wrinkles and increase elasticity, but also to improve your health and well being!

Whether you are Pre-Menopausal or Menopausal the secret to aging skin and youthful skin is found right here! Hydration! Why do we lose this as we age? A baby's body weight is 75% water. An adult's weight is composed of 50 % water. The main reason for this as we get older, our cells break down and gradually lose our ability to absorb and lock in water. As this happens we lose the smooth firm and supple skin we once had as a youth.

If you are tired of rough skin, wrinkles and want more smoothness and hydration, please read on. You may be old or young, but you aren't what you feel, and I will help you to feel emotionally and physically better than you have in years!

Over my 30 years as a practicing Esthetician and a successful Day Spa owner I have come to realize that everything I do to help people renew rejuvenate and protect their skin is based on two main principles: Maintain the barrier function of the skin, and to help the skin hold as much moisture as possible. The next paragraphs will be on the events that occur within the skin as we age that truly affect the skin barriers function and its ability to hold water.

Your Top Layer of Skin (Excerpts from Dr. Howard Murad)

Throughout life the constant turnover of dead cells that rests on top of the epidermis doesn't change much. Studies have shown that this layer thins with age, but it remains protective, and if well cared for will adequately prevent moisture loss from the layers beneath it. Dead cells tend to linger longer as you age hence older skin feels rougher than younger skin.

Pigment Production
(Excerpts from Dr.Murad)

Skin contains pigment to protect it from the Sun. The cells that produce this pigment are known as melanin. They make up about 3% of your cells in the epidermis. Each melanin cell is called a melanocyte, and provides melanin for about 36 skin cells. The number of active melaninocytes decreases by an estimated 10-20% per decade of your adult life. The melanocytes that remain attempt to compensate for the missing ones, hence you have an overproduction of pigment that occurs in one area and a decline in one area or a complete absence in another. This is why age spots form and your skin becomes very dark and light shades of color.

Infection Fighters
Excerpts (from Dr. Howard Murad)

The reason we are seeing more skin cancer and infection is that as we age, the Langerhan's cells decrease, and they are found in the epidermis and are major players in the skins immune response. According to health estimates, as much as half of Langerhans cells are lost by late adulthood, which may explain why older skin is very susceptible to infection and skin cancer.

Skin Anchors
(Excerpts from Dr. Howard Murad)

These are age related changes. When the epidermis meets the dermis. Over times these straight tissues flatten, and the two no longer share nutrients as they once did. They are not tightly attached as they once were, and a minor injury can separate them. That is why Post-Menopausal skin blisters or bleeds more easily than younger skin.

Blood Vessels (Capillaries)

With aging blood vessels that carry nutrients and moisture to the skin begin to diminish; Sun damage makes the vessels even worse. It causes the walls to thicken, and eventually as they dilate you can now see them. They look and appear on the skins surface as tiny red threads, hence broken capillaries.

Moisture holds Molecules (Excerpts by Dr. Howard Murad)

The matrix of fibers in the dermis is built upon collagen and elastin. The molecules contained in these fibers are called Gags. They are water loving molecules that keep everything moist, and moisture is the secret to keeping everything in the skin collagen and elastin pliable. Over time this collagen and elastin is lost and with sun exposure it doubles with time.

Collagen and Elastin Fibers

Most of the signs of aging begin in the tough fibrous dermis of your skin. Collagen and Elastin form the skin's infrastructure and give it strength and resiliency. With aging, the number of fibroblasts that make the two-decrease and skin repair begins to slow down.

(Excerpt from Dr. Howard Murad)

In fact, it was aging researcher Leonard Hayflicks experiments with fibroblasts from the skin of fetuses in the early 60's that led to one of the widely accepted theories of why we age. Hayflicks discovered that our cells divide a predictable and infinite number of times and when they stop, we age! Wrinkles begin forming years before they are etched in the skin, or before the force of gravity becomes obvious. Some of the cellular changes are part of the inevitable slow down that occurs throughout the body. But another factor that occurs is caused by sunlight and emotional or harsh treatment to the skin. That seems to be the first basis for wrinkling of the skin.

Smoking is one harsh treatment that causes your skin to age. Nicotine causes the blood vessels to contract, so less oxygen bearing blood reaches the skin. By bending the collagen repeatedly it creates bends and it breaks therefore resulting in permanent wrinkles.

Aging causes an increase in enzymes that eat up collagen and elastin fibers. As they age we no longer produce enough D.N.A. to allow the cells to divide as quickly and efficiently as they once did. By the time you turn 70 or 80, you now have clusters of these sluggish old cells deep within the skin. At 25 or 35 years of age you probably had none.

These cells don't just hang around; they are destructive because they churn out collagen chewing enzymes. One reason that wrinkles form is that collagen and elastin fibers are being destroyed and repair of the fibers has slowed considerably. The fibroblasts are greatly diminishing as well. The damage that is done over the years is probably why cells in our skin decline. The damage is caused by several forces, and that is why we have to understand how we can help the skin to rejuvenate and recouped during the times of menopause and post- menopause.

The most important tip that you must remember to help the aging process is water. Moisture keeps the skin healthy, luminous, and strikingly beautiful!

Your skin is your body's protective envelope and protecting it is your main objective. Toxic chemicals, pollutants, ultraviolet radiation, sunlight, and many agents that cause inflammation form free radicals within the skin.

Your job is continuing maintenence and repair of your only skin that you have until you die! Though keeping up with your skin may sound boring, it is the only skin you will have for the rest of your life and only you can keep it healthy! So let us get to work on how to look vibrant and feel better!

My anti-aging formula is quite simple. Whether you are oily, dry, combination skin or just plain sensitive- you must follow the same principles every day and night. Your skin cells will want to perform at their top level. The healthier your skin is, the better able it is to cope with hormonal ups and downs, time, sun, and stress of life.

With any skin, your job is to keep it very clean, hydrated, nourished, and to make it more resilient to nature's enemies.In the morning use a cleanser that is rich in skin soothers followed by a hydrating toner. If oily, use a deep pore cleanser to wash skin followed by a pore purifying astringent. Then while the skin is still moist and dewy, give it a boost of antioxidants to combat free radicals that are in the environment. Then you seal in all these radical fighters with a light vitamin enriched moisturizer. Whether you are oily, you can use my shine- free moisturizer or you can use my moisture rich crème for dry skin, you are supplying important hydration. Then apply your sun block over these ingredients or buy a moisturizer with a sun block contained in the product such as Dr.Murad's Environmental Defense or his Resurgence Line for Menopausal clients. I also have Skin Lines specifically meant for Menopause, Rosacea, Sensitive, and Oily Skins.

Your sun block should always be oil-free so that you do not develop whiteheads in the t-zone area, and a SPF 15 or more is suggested, whether you live in Chicago or in Florida. Your next step should be to apply eye protection to the top of your lids as well as the under layer of your eye. Eye Gelee can be used for puffiness and for oily skin, and eye firming crème can be used for evening to hydrate and nourish the area.

There is also an eye cream by Dr. Murad that has a SPF15 contained in the crème if you would like protection during the day.

Once or twice a week exfoliate with a light grainy product such as Refining Grains, or my Chamomile Scrub or Peppermint Scrub for Oily Skin. Once to twice a week you should apply a mask to help keep oil flow down, or to hydrate and moisturize. I have a wonderful masque that helps to alleviate oil flow in the t-zone area called Vita plus Masque, and it is also excellent for dry and sensitive skins as it helps to take down redness and moisturize the neck and décolleté area.

Once a week it is good to give yourself an Alpha Hyrdroxy Treatment for problem skin, or dehydrated skin as it takes the top layer of your skin and gently exfoliates as well as hydrates the skin. It shocks the top layer and helps to keep it more resilient and luminous.

Night Crèmes are very important in any type of skin. There are two reasons for this. One is loss of water during the evening, and it is greatest at night. Two- the body's cells are replenished with nutrients and natural plant extracts to give your skin a chance to rejuvenate and hydrate. I have a wonderful night crème that is called Endurance Age Control Crème and it has chamomile, green tea, allantoin, and aloe to soothe as well as to hydrate. For an oily skin, I have a product called Shine Free Solution that will cut your oil flow in half during the night time.

With every type of skin, this formula is necessary and will be altered according to skin type, season, and sensitivity to products.

A good Esthetician will be able to determine what skin type, pore type, hydration test, and skin care regime is needed for any skin type, and will cater your Facial and regime to accommodate your skin care concerns.

With hormones lessening, you will find a plentitude of problems associated with your skin due to hormone fluctuation or lack thereof.

One problem is hyper pigmentation, and can be found after the birth of a baby, too much sun, or simply from driving your car with the sun beating down on the side of your face or hands. The pigment signs of aging start to appear and the best solution for this problem is a Hydroquinone product lined with a sun block of 15 or more to keep the skin protected from the environment. In our Facial room we have a prelightening process that we use to lighten the darkened area up to two shades lighter, and it is then up to you to follow this regime at home with a product that you can apply morning and night before your moisturizer. Note: Pregnant or lactating women cannot have our prelightening treatment or the Hydroquinone product applied until they are through with this passage, as studies have not been completely shown to be safe for the unborn child.

Menopausal skin has its own problems as well. Besides losing collagen fibers and elastisicity, you will find hair growing in the most unlikely places...areas you never thought a hair could grow, it does! Then to top this off, your eyebrows thin and your hair on the top of your head go through maximum changes! Waxing or Laser Hair Removal is strongly suggested during this time, because as you age the hairs become coarser and thicker on your face and neck area, and lessen in other areas such as your underarms and bikini line. I have found white hairs on my chin area, and I swear it has happened over night while I slept!

Women that have never had breakouts in their life may find that they develop hormone breakouts such as pimples or worse yet, a developing problem called Rosacea that causes sensitivity, redness, breakouts, and enlarged pore size. This problem can be solved with a good Rosacea Facial combined with a proper skin care regime, and healthy habits on the patient's part to help alleviate stress, caffeine, sun, and alcohol levels to keep the Rosacea at a minimum. If this regime does not work for the patient, we then send the patient to a good dermatologist for their help in solving this problem. As we age, we develop thinner skin, and more sensitive skin and I find Rosacea a common problem during this passage of time.

Sensitive skin becomes more prevalent, and what used to work for you when you were younger does not play a part in Menopausal skin! Skin cell turnover is very sluggish, wrinkles are starting to form around your eye and face area, and you just need more hydration and a little shock therapy by a good Esthetician to wake up this top layer of skin and hydrate it! A good Algae Treatment, A Vitamin C Treatment, Microdermabrasion Treatment are all suggestions that you could get to rejuvenate your skin and also bring more hydration back to the upper layers. You will leave a Salon with your skin luminous and glowing, as well as clean and rehydrated.

Just a little more about Rosacea-In my practice I find more women developing this skin condition. Ten years ago, it was virtually unheard of, and now I find 2 out of 10 patients age 40-65 with this condition. Of course when I entered Peri- Menopause I developed this condition. I had rosacea for the last 7 years and now that I am in Menopause, it has subsided quite a bit. I do believe that part of this condition is due in part to a woman's hormones fluctuating up and down so rapidly, combined with extreme stress in their life and a genetic background of sensitivity. My clinical studies show that after the age of 65 and menopause ceases, Rosacea seems to take a back seat to dehydration, and those pores finally calm down!

If after Rosacea Facials do not help, then a good Dermatologist is in order to take a good look at your skin, and probably put you on a gel or crème for Rosacea and possibly antibiotics for a period of time. I prefer to take the natural approach and work with my own line of Rosacea products, as well as Dr. Murad's Rosacea Line, they are excellent at calming the skin down.

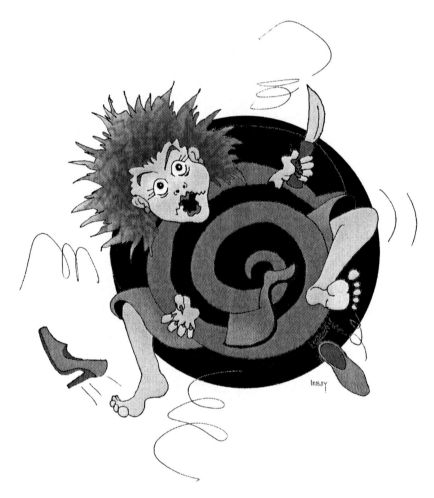

Crazy, Hostile?

That's not me!!

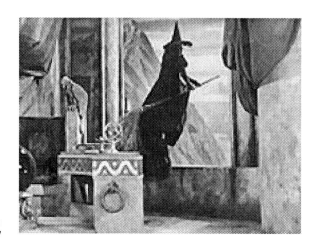

Chapter 12

Case studies of Peri-Menopausal, Menopausal, and Post-Menopausal Women – Hey, That's Me

By Linda LaVelle A.T.I.E. I.T.E.C.

I am a woman in menopause for the last four years, and my life has truly changed since the onset of this menace. I have been moody, temperamental, judgmental, and at many times uncontrollable with emotion. I have learned to control my moods with positive thinking, weight training and exercise, the will to survive an alien inside my body and brain, and the power of prayer. I have been through 25 hot flashes a day, many night sweats in the evening, clothes ripping off and nightgowns going back on. "Blonde Bitch" was my name for one or two years, and bloated was how I felt every day while forgetting where I was and what I was going there for! Heart palpitations was a common everyday occurrence, and the scariest event for me, anxiety attacks when you least expect them not to mention lack of sleep the real reason why I can write this book at 3 A.M.!

The one thing that I have learned about this passage in life is there are at least 25 things that can go wrong with you, and medicine is not black and white. No one doctor has the right answer for everyone; you must gather all your information and make the decision that you feel is best for you.

There are many ways to make pizza and you must find the right recipe for yourself and judge what tastes best for you!

I am truly a testament to surviving the onslaught of menopause. You cannot take this passage of life lying down. You have to educate yourself on the subject, read as much as you can on your choices, and decide what's right for you and your body. I did not want to lose the woman that I had become before Menopause and I can truly say that I valiantly fought the enemy until I won the war!

You have choices and many options, so I give you examples of several stories of real women experiencing the same thing as I have, so that you can make up your own mind and decide what is right for you!

It takes commitment to approach this time of life with grace, anticipation, and a real willingness to look at the real you inside of yourself not just emotionally, but physically as well.

I can only speak for my age group, but I do know that each passage of life brings its rewards if you know what you want in life. I was looking for peace, serenity, good health, and more sexiness. If this might interest you, then by all means please read on!

I must warn you, you have to have a positive attitude during this passage of life, and you must have the willingness to go through many trials of menopause before finding the right choice for you. You must decide if you should go natural replacement, bio-identical hormone, or synthetic hormones. What ever choice you make, you must embrace it with a positive attitude and be the confident and balanced woman that you have prayed for!

You have choices and many options, so I will now give you some examples of several stories from real women experiencing the same thing as I have, then you can make up your own mind and decide exactly what is right for you! I have decided to change the names of my cases with Hurricane names. I live in South Florida, the land of vicious weather in the summertime, and when I asked my friends and family what they likened a hurricane to; they commonly described a woman going into menopause with out a doubt! Here are some of the descriptions that they gave for a hurricane and you can decide for yourself! A nuisance, a mess, nothing but anxiety and trouble, a wild wind, very temperamental, unpredictable, goes in circles and then comes right back again, and finally...and uncontrollable force! We are now in "La Nina" so please read on to see my girls in their hurricane passage of life!

Arlene 35-40 Years Old - P.M.S.

Arlene has P.M.S at its most high! She has regular periods and she is a highly charged woman, sexual as well as mental. All week long she struggles to maintain a healthy balance between the employees she works with, and the husband that she loves. Most of the time she gets into gigantic arguments with both and ends up wanting to punch somebody out!

During her week before her period, she becomes electrically charged; she fights with everyone including her dog, and literally tells her husband to take it and shove it or his life is history! She finally gets back to herself about the 3rd day of her period after bloating and heavy bleeding ceases. After her period, she is back on her electrically charged treadmill fighting to be Arlene again.

From my viewpoint it is a fight for flight syndrome and she is just starting! Her hormonal balance is jumping up and down like a roller coaster, and it seems to have taken charge of her life physically and mentally and emotionally.

Arlene has gained 10 to 15 pounds since she got married nearly 3 years ago. She is a perfectionist by nature, and her job as well as her family life reflects this .She tries to be the best cook and wife that she can. However her life does not go as she plans, and she becomes very short tempered, and always looking for a fight!

When Arlene and her husband first married, they lived in cramped quarters the first two years of their married life. They found their dream home and were slowly remodeling the house of their dreams when along came two hurricanes and destroyed what was remodeled. The stress of a new marriage, remodeling, hurricanes, working hard at her profession, being the perfect wife, and helping out with many family problems had taken a toll on Arlene.

Never did Arlene realize that she was out of whack hormonally. Nor did she realize that she might need hormone replacement at this time of her life. From a skin specialist's viewpoint, I could see that her adrenal glands were overworking. Her skin is extremely oily. She breaks out constantly and emotionally she is heading for a big crash!

Her husband is very loving and understanding. He allows her to be herself and pitches in to help her with household chores and needed items for the house. Her main complaint is that he is a "pest "and that he let things go too easily without a fight. She complains that he "knows it all" and she constantly tries to show him that he's not right all the time! Her life is electrically charged and maybe you relate to the way Arlene feels. She does not want to lose her marriage nor her job, and she wants to work on herself and her addiction to perfection .She is going to go to her gynecologist and have a full panel run of her hormones and see just what she is lacking in this highly charged emotional state of mind. Does this sound like you?

Charley 47 Years Old – Perimenopausal

One week before her period Charley cries over spilled water. She hates her life, she always wants to quit her wonderful and fulfilling job as a lawyer, and she wants to move out of her beautiful home. She has a wonderful son, a gratifying job that pays very well, money in her savings and 401(k), a house that is fully paid for, a car that is brand new and she really doesn't have to work if she doesn't feel the need, and yet she is unhappy with her life! On her cell phone for old boyfriends, she has "scum of the earth" and "nut job" for responses! The scary thing is that she just might talk to these fools if the mood is right...

She gets very irritated if you suggest anything out of her "ordinary". She can't make any normal decisions, and crisscrosses back on her decisions that she has made. Just try to shop with her! She will take back half of the things that she buys, and it's not because they are not cute or pretty, she just can't make up her mind! Her periods are getting light. She is on thyroid medication for an overactive thyroid, and she fights the mental stress of a single mother with no help from a partner. She has become very independent and willing to cope with whatever comes her way. Charley is very emotional and unavailable at times, leaving the phone off the hook if she is in that mood!

Psychologically she seems to be avoiding the next step that is coming. That step is not being able to cope with menopause and the feelings that come with it. . She will not be a fertile woman anymore; some sort of punishment must be involved with this passage of life! There is a week in her month where she wants to be locked in a closet until it is all over. She is very temperamental, wanting solitude, and longing for a partner just to love and tell her troubles to.

Once a month when I do her facial I find that her skin is becoming more sensitive to ingredients, and her moisture level is dropping, becoming drier. Being of Mediterranean influence her aging is minimal, but I do find that when her thyroid drops, her skin gets drier and the texture of her skin changes as well as her coloring of her skin from a pale beige to a more sallow color.

At this time of her life she needs an update from her gynecologist on what hormones she is temporarily lacking; what she needs emotionally, as well as what her body is telling her only her gynecologist can help her out with these decisions. Does this sound like you?

Frances 50 Years Old - Menopausal

Francis has been in menopause now for almost 1 year, her periods have ceased, and she is afraid to take any form of medication to help relieve her menopausal symptoms. After the scare two to three years ago, she decided to brave it out and what has evolved is not a pretty sight!

She is lucky if she sleeps five hours a night. She has many night sweats and she prefers to sleep nude at night. It doesn't really matter if she does sleep nude. She is not very interested in having sex at this time of her life.

When I give Francis her facial, I find very dry skin, redness of the nose and cheek area due to broken capillary veins, and aging and thinning of the skin due to severe sun damage and her lack of hormones.

She tells me of extreme dryness in the vagina area as well as many hot flashes through out the day. Talk about a woman on extreme edge. She feels like an alien is inside her body and has invaded it, while she just sits on the sidelines just watching her life go by.

One morning Frances was sitting at the breakfast nook just waking up and having her first cup of coffee. Her husband Bob is a prominent attorney in town, and he just walked into the kitchen area with his briefcase ready to start his day. He tripped on his shoelace, dropped his briefcase to the ground, and knocked her off her chair along with her coffee! Now anyone else would react with a laugh, but not Francis...She picks up her coffee cup, throws the cup at Bob, yells at what an idiot he is, throws him out of the kitchen and locks the back door! She is so enraged at him that she won't let him back in the kitchen, and poor Bob just wants to go to work! She starts screaming at him through the back door that she is sick of him and she wants a divorce and please get the hell out of her life! Poor Bob, he just wants his briefcase that is lying on the kitchen floor and can't wait to get to work so he can be in his own little world away from this holy terror that has gone temporarily insane! Bob starts pleading with his wife to please just give him his briefcase so that he can get the hell out of this horrible situation gone bad, and now the neighbors are hearing the fight, and he just wants to crawl to his car, briefcase or not!

Within five to 10 minutes she comes to her senses, lets him back in and apologizes for her behavior. She tells Bob that she really loves him and that he has been very patient and understanding but having an alien invades her mind and body is just too much for her to tolerate. She is definitely a woman on the edge of a hormonal breakdown all due to her lack of hormones. She feels dead inside and her vibration of living is virtually gone. Her memory loss is rapidly accelerating and she forgets her appointments with me as well as her appointments for her teenage son. She can't find her glasses, and she forgets to go to the dry cleaners, leaving her money at home, and leaving her son waiting at the High School! When a woman reaches menopause, it causes more women to be overly aggressive and left without that soft clear thinking that a woman on hormones will have.

Francis definitely needs to see her doctor or gynecologist for an updated test on her hormone level, so that she can make some decisions in her life .Does this sound like you?

Ivana 53 Years Old - Menopausal

Ivana has been in menopause since the age of 50. She was very afraid of hormone therapy and was always going to great lengths to try a natural regime. She had been trying black cohosh, soy capsules, estroven for hot flashes, and progesterone cream from her local pharmacy. She was on a variety of natural vitamins that included calcium, vitamin C and vitamin E. She was even taking Sex Again! A pill that is supposed to bring your sex life back to normal!

She had been trying everything out of the ordinary hoping to restore her hormones and when this regime did not work she came in to see me for a facial. She started crying over the fact that she hated her husband who is a prominent doctor in town and she hated her 18-year-old son that can't wait to turn 21. She wants to kick the boy out, and the husband wants her to find her own apartment, so that she can find her own self! Ivana knows that there is something wrong with her life…she is a bitchy, temperamental, judgmental, hot sweating holy mother of God mess!!

When I last saw Ivana she was very afraid of hormone therapy and had gained about 10 pounds. When I did her facial, I noticed that her skin had started a condition called rosacea and this had increased on her nose and cheek area. Her skin moisture level was extremely dry and she was starting the thinning of the skin and deep age lines around her eye area. Upon looking at her skin, I found the extreme dryness with the lack of clear color. Her pigmentation had become very blotchy due in part to sun damage and lowered estrogen hormones. I wanted to pre-lighten her skin with vitamin C and glycolic acid to give her a lighter skin tone and increase her hydration level. Ivana has many hairs starting on her chin and lip area. Her hairs have been getting darker and with more frequency. I also find skin tags appearing on her neck and décolleté area with frequency. She seems to be taking on a pear shaped appearance from what was a size 6 figure. She claims her mother never had menopause this bad, and she just does not know where to turn to. Does this sound like you?

Wilma 54 Years Old - Menopausal

I wanted to save the best for the last. I am writing from my home without light and air conditioning, the gusty winds are now ending. It was the scariest, frightening hurricane that I have ever been through. The good thing is the weather will change dramatically from summer to fall as soon as Wilma is out to sea. We will experience 50-60 degree weather for the next few days allowing us to survey the damage that is truly immense around us. I am sure glad that I have my hormones in check as I was starting to hyperventilate when Wilma was on her way over to the east coast and was a Category 2 with 120 mph winds. This morning I woke to frogs jumping in my family room, crickets singing their songs, and lizards leaping from the plants that we had stored everywhere. Last night, I held a fight with ants crawling under my family room carpet from the outside plants that were stored in back of my couches, and a few wasps flying around as I envisioned their last fly by as I killed them with exactness. Never could I have dealt with this hurricane had I not been in check with my hormones! I had a husband marching through the rooms during the hurricane checking any interior damage, and jumping at us periodically. I had my son lying next to me on the bed with his ADHD kicking me and asking me when the worst would be over. The dog was crawling all over my body begging for this ordeal to be over, and the wind howling through our house with the screened in porch that we just replaced breathing in and out. It was truly the storm from Hell, and now we are in its aftermath. The lights are out, the phone doesn't work, the air conditioning is bye-bye for a few days, and thank God I bought enough food to make hamburgers out on the grill, and shrimp on the Barbie plus plenty of wine and cheese to take care of the whole neighborhood! Do you see, my hormones are in check, and I am dealing with life as it comes! This is the most awesome thing as the last hurricane that occurred, I hated my husband, I wanted a divorce and he was the most uncontrollable force in my life at that time. In retrospect, I see that it was partially me who was intense with craziness at the time, and it was hard for him to deal with my emotions as well as his. But this hurricane is different! I have my strong constitution back again, and I have no depression in place, as well as a feeling of loneliness. I am so grateful to be alive and well with my family in place and with all prayers that encompassed this horrible hurricane my house and family was unscathed! I don't know about our businesses however we will survey that tomorrow and pray for God's graces upon that scenario. I just wanted to prove to you that with proper hormones your life is in proper check with everyone else around you, and you are like your fellow neighbors... happy to be alive and well and with house attached despite a horrible hurricane!

So I beg of you, go and get your hormones checked by your Gynecologist as the more people that I talk to, they are unhappy with their lives, they want a new husband or lover, and they want a new everything... Only you can do the tests, and it takes a positive attitude towards life, and a willingness to cope with whatever comes your way to get through this passage in life. But with hormones in check, you can do it! So go forth, and be proud of yourself for forging ahead on your being your own woman!

Jeanne 57 Years Old - Menopausal

Jeanne has been in menopause since 51 years of age. She has suffered from irregular sleeping patterns since the onset of menopause. When she went to her doctor, he gave her Premarin at the onset of menopause, but when the scare came out about HT, she threw them out in the garbage. She was very afraid of trying any new hormonal therapy.

Jeannie has been married for 24 years to a man that is 10 years older than her. They have not had sex in seven years, and she adores her husband but he does not give her the romantic love that she feels is missing in her marriage. She told me a story about one incident that was sad but funny! Her mother had just died, and she was going to the funeral with her daughter and her grandson. They were stranded on the way home to Florida by bad weather and airline difficulties. They were staying in a small hotel room with very little sleep. When morning came Jeanne woke up quietly and was going to start the little coffee pot. Her daughter was blow drying her hair in the bathroom and her grandson was just waking up. As Jeanne turns on the little light to start the coffee going, her grandson jumps up out of bed and screams to his grandmother "turn that damn light off" and tells his grandmother to be more quiet! She always defended her grandson thinking he was such a good little boy, and now he is telling her to shut up and turn the damn light off! She jumps over to him as well as her daughter, and they both are ready to strangle him! The daughter is hitting him with the brush yelling "don't talk to your Grandma like that" Of course the grandson says sarcastically "oh you're really killing me Grandma"! As they are all screaming at each other, the bill gets thrown under the hotel room door and they all stop screaming for fear that they will get reported to the authorities for child abuse! They went on to the airplane with no one talking to each other for hours. That incident scared Jeanne as she did not realize that her emotions had overtaken her clear mind! When she got back to Florida, she made an appointment with her Gynecologist, as she felt like her anger was getting out of control. Jeanne thought she might need stronger hormone therapy to help regulate some of her anger. She is presently using estrogen cream from the Medicine Shop without a Doctors prescription, and she also uses progesterone cream 14 days out of each month. She uses testosterone tablets called sexy ones and swears that it is so powerful she has no need for them anymore so she gave them to me! I of course tried them for one month with no luck at all!

Jeannie has found herself a lover and sees him once a month when he arrives in town. She swears that her sex life has never been more fulfilling, and she does not want to give him up! Her sexual libido is alive and well, but her vagina is drying up! Jeanne also buys K.Y Jelly to help alleviate her dryness and vaginal irritation. She worries that her husband may find out about this affair, but she is willing to let this happen just to keep the love affair going on, and so far he does not suspect a thing, so the torrid love affair will continue without interruption!

Upon inspection of Jeannie's skin, I find that melasma is developing from the sun as well as her lack of estrogen in her body. She breaks out hormonally on her chin and her cheeks. Her hairs are growing rapidly on her chin and sides of her face. When I see Jeanne for her facial, I wax her face and chin area, before performing the deep cleansing of the skin. Jeannie's dietary habits are nutritionally correct, however at night she enjoys drinking her wine and not drinking enough water, which creates dryness of the skin. In the last six months, she has also noticed the weight gain of approximately 10 to 15 pounds. Jeannie has a pear shaped figure and she worries that she cannot seem to lose the weight that she has recently accumulated. She will go on a detox diet for one or two days, and then go off of the diet in the evening when 5:00 wine coolers start!

Jeannie's mental clarity seems to be normal, and her sex life with her lover seems to be going well. Her one main complaint is that she is not able to sleep all night like she used to. She still has night sweats one or two times a night, and she still has to rip her nightgown on and off before she can fall asleep. I suggested that she go to her gynecologist for an update on her hormones and get a complete blood work up.

After seeing Jeannie last month, her husband of 24 years has asked for a divorce as he found out about her lover and she is very devastated and confused. Her lover says that he will still be by her side, but that he also has a wife and two children who are not raised completely, and does not want to leave them. She feels lost and confused and I told her that if she sees her doctor he will help her to sleep better and to feel better about herself emotionally. Does this sound like you?

Katrina 60 Years Old - Menopausal

Katrina has been in menopause for almost ten years now. She has been on a hormone replacement called Premarin for the last five years. Her gynecologist has suggested that she be placed on hormone replacement therapy for the next 10 years. She is a happy, well centered woman and she has the energy of a woman in her forties! She watches her diet; she takes many nutrients and drinks plenty of water daily. She claims her sex life has never been better with her husband of 35 years.

Katrina has been in a real estate business with her husband and family, and does not want to retire. Her husband and her family are in the business with Katrina and she actually run circles around her family! She wants to work until she no longer can and as far as I can see; her mental clarity and her strength and vitality will keep her going strong!

Upon examination of Katrina's skin, I found a skin of a forty year old woman with occasional breakouts in the t-zone area, no noticeable melasma and a thicker skin like a younger woman not in her 60's! Katrina has very few wrinkles as well as fine lines and she takes extreme care of her skin. She watches her skin like she watches her body! I have never met anyone that has her spunk and her energy. I really admire her and hope that I can be like her when I am in my 60s!

Katrina has had a face lift and a tummy tuck, but I think that Katrina would still look great even without the plastic surgery; she is just that type of woman. I can honestly say that she is one of the few women I know that have her hormones in place and it really shows! She is vibrant full of life beautiful inside and out how and very sexy! Does this sound like you? (You can only hope that this is how you will be in your 60s!)

Ophelia 72 years Old - Post Menopausal

Ophelia has been post menopausal for over 10 years, and she can't seem to remember the exact time when she entered menopause but she thinks that it was in her early 50's when she lived up north. One cold wintry night in Chicago she remembers vividly making her husband keep the bedroom window open as she was having a night sweat or hot flash. He put a baseball cap on, a pair of sweats over his pajamas and a pair of heavy socks on for warmth. They proceeded to go to sleep in the frigid bedroom. Ophelia recalls never sleeping better that night, and even through the night sweats and the night gown going off and on, the window remained open all night. When Ophelia woke in the morning, her husband looks at her and says "do you see the pile of snow by the window. Do you think it is cold enough for you now??" He then told her to go and see her doctor and figure out what is wrong with her! Ophelia never wanted to talk about it with her husband, but she remembers discussing it with her girlfriend and they both agree it was a time riddled with fights, crying, and lack of understanding from their mates.

Ophelia remembers going to her Gynecologist and he put her on Premarin for menopause symptoms and she felt wonderful for many years until the scare came from the media about H.R.T and cancer! That ended her hormone therapy as she stopped taking her pills at 69 years of age. Her night sweats came back gradually and her vaginal dryness was intolerable. She swears that she lost an inch from her height and she has been having trouble with extreme dryness in her skin and thinning of her hair.

Upon examination of Ophelia's skin, I found age lines of a normal 70 year old woman, her elasticity and tone was lacking of moisture, and sagging of the lower part of the face was evident. The firmness of her skin had started to decrease over the last few years, and she has been complaining about the skin starting to fall. Ophelia works out by walking daily, golfing 2-3 times a week and taking multivitamins with calcium. Her doctor has recently put her on Fosamax to help increase her bone density and she does not want to lose any more inches of height than she has already!

Ophelia drinks plenty of water during the day with her exercise regime, but I know at night she likes to have her martinis with her husband at dinner or with friends when they entertain on weekends.

Ophelia has a very busy life as a retiree and so long as her husband keeps his busy pace with his friends during the day and she gets to be with her girlfriends playing bridge or golf it is a fulfilling life for her even without her hormonal therapy. She still seems to have good mental clarity and maintain a wonderful sense of humor.

Ophelia wants to keep her skin and body in excellent shape, so she opts for monthly facials and regular Microdermabrasion treatments as well as Sea Salt Glow treatments for her dehydrated skin. We are definitely making headway in the aging process and halting the long term effects of sun and wrinkles!

Does Ophelia sound like you?

Patricia 78 Years Old - Post Menopausal

Patricia is one of the most well balanced postmenopausal women I have ever met! She just sold her business of 25 years for 5 million dollars and is worrying about her capital gains that she is going to accumulate. She is presently training the new owners on the business she has worried and fretted over for all those years! She has met a wonderful man her age after losing her husband to cancer 2 years previously and wants to move in with him and start a new life together in a new home! They will be unified, yet not complete as a married couple for they have family to contend with and many grandchildren that are contained in trust accounts that they are worried about! They are moving in together in non –wedded bliss and to happily share their lives together.

Before she met her recent partner, she was dating five men at one time! She was always afraid of all of the men meeting at once, so she took great pains to keep them all at a distance. One lover lived in Georgia, one lived in San Francisco, one lived in New York, and one lived in Tampa. The fifth one lived right in her town of Stuart, Florida. When I would see Patricia for her Facial and Microderm treatment, I would get dizzy just hearing about how she would juggle these men around and they not run into each other! Patricia was very afraid of emotional attachment to any one man, and so she would go to great pains to keep all of her men! One weekend she would see the Stuart man, then the next weekend she would fly to New York and see N.Y. man, and the one man in San Francisco she would only see twice a year as he would only come in to town for business meetings. Where the trouble came in was the man in Stuart and the man in Tampa... they were all vying for her attention and wanted to be the only one in her life. All five men knew that she had other interests, and she had clearly stated to all that she had no interest in getting serious with anyone. The surprise came one summer day when she was rushed to a Hospital with pains in her chest. It turned out to be heart problems, and a bypass was suggested with a long stay at home for recuperation. This literally changed her life, as now she saw which man was truly in love with her, and it was the Stuart man! He stayed with her during the hospital stay as well as the nights at home, and had it not been for Bob and his loving care she would not be here to tell me this story! He acted like a devoted husband doting on her every need! That is when she decided to get rid of all the other men in her life and just be unified with Bob!

Upon examination of her skin, I can't get over the fact that her skin has remained so firm and tight. Patricia had a face lift when she turned 60, but I truly believe that with her Celtic skin tone she should have aged long before her time. I questioned her about her hormones, and she said that she had been taking synthetic hormones since the age of 38 years, as she had a complete hysterectomy and was advised to go on hormone therapy after the surgery. Her gynecologist was instrumental in keeping her vitality and strength in her face and body. Her bone density is that of a 50 year old woman, and her ability to maintain her clarity of mind as well as her sanity is well acknowledged! I strongly believe that without her hormone therapy she would not look or feel as well as she does! You definitely want to be like Patricia at age 78! Does this sound like you?

Rita 58 Years Old - Menopausal

Rita is a strange exception to many menopausal and post menopausal women. When Rita found out that I was writing a book on Menopause, she called my Spa to tell me that she has never had any side effects associated with this passage in life. Rita is a vibrant energetic woman and very happily married to a corporate developer for over 25 years now. I admire Rita's tenacity and her strength and strong attitude towards life and its struggles, but I can honestly tell you that she is of the 25% of women that have not suffered with one ill effect from Menopause.

I have not examined her skin as she comes to my Day Spa for other services, however from an outward view she seems to be aging slowly. Her skin seems to be of good thick texture, and her moisture level seems to be of normal nature, that being 35%. She drinks at least 8 glasses of water daily, and takes daily doses of multi-vitamins. Rita's hair and her eyebrows have not thinned out as most menopausal women have experienced. Rita has started the sagging progression of her skin and jowl area. Rita has not had a face lift and does not want any plastic surgery.

Rita's genetics have definitely played an important role in how she feels and how mild her menopause symptoms have been. I certainly applaud her for how well she has gone through this passage in life and without a complaint!

Does this sound like you? If so, you are the fortunate woman!!

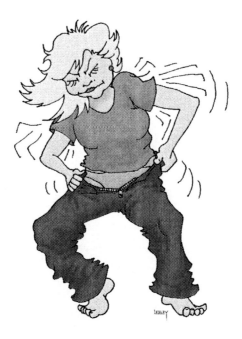

When your new jeans just don't fit anymore!

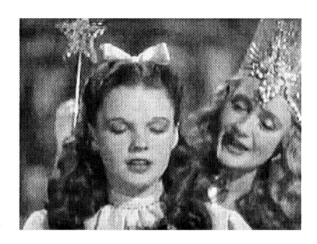

Chapter 13

Nutritional Therapy, Diet, and Exercise- Now I'm Feeling Better than Ever!

By Linda LaVelle A.T.I.E. I.T.E.C.

When it comes to how you feel, hormonal balance is everything. Your hormones when in proper balance make you feel at your peak; wonderful, optimistic, energetic, keen and very sexy!

When your hormones are not in balance, fighting physical aging becomes harder to achieve than ever before. Finding balance allows us to forget all the symptoms that were plaguing us before menopause.

I have decided to take charge of my body and do something about this problem. I focus on how great I look for my age. I never thought that I would look this good at 54 years of age. One of the big advantages is that we now know how to take care of ourselves better than our parents did. We understand nutrition better than ever before and as women we really understand the benefits of exercise. For example, weight training in particular promotes bone growth. When you are lifting weights the muscles tug against the bone, promoting and increasing the bone growth. Your physical and emotional benefits are seen immediately.

Nothing is more beautiful than toned, defined and cut muscles. Your clothes will look better on you, you will be in a clothing size you only imagined and the most exciting part is that you will be building bone mass. In a case where there is bone loss you will be restoring bone and creating a serotonin level that will leave you energized all day long!

One of the most important things I've found that would help my serotonin level to peak was to go for a weekly exercise regime that included three days of extensive weight training (30 minutes) followed by a 30 minute cardiovascular workout. I started this at age 49 and have continued this routine well into my 50's. I started with a personal trainer, but you can just join a local gym and they will orient you with the equipment and give you a routine for your physique. I found I have more energy and I can face the day of hard work ahead of me much more effectively and with more optimism.

The most important thing to be concerned with when you are training is your diet. My personal trainer constantly stressed that 90 percent of your work out regime consists of a diet low in carbohydrates and high in protein. For the first month, no dairy products, pasta, bread of any sort or sugar. After the first three months I lost 15 pounds and by the sixth month I had lost another 10 pounds. I was down to a size 6 which has always had been a dream of mine!

Then a tragedy came my way. I had a car accident and was no longer able to work out like I used to, no weight training, just walking and light swimming. I was then gaining weight rapidly. My high protein diet was not sustaining my healthy trim body any longer. I realized two things were happening, my hormones were out of whack and it was very hard to stay slim like I used to. I was starting to look like my mother, stomach increasing, legs getting flabby and my body sliding down the mountain! I was becoming insulin resistant, which explains why it gets harder to stay slim as you get older.

Adopting a high carbohydrate diet exacerbates the problem, because all of those carbohydrates increase insulin resistance. The elevated amount of insulin in the blood increases testosterone levels, which decreased the production of estrogen and progesterone, the female sex hormones. Compound that with a low fat diet and you have less of a hormone production. I've found that you need dietary fat to create hormones. The uncomfortable side effects of hot flashes, night sweats, mood swings, memory loss and imbalance of these sex hormones means that we cannot produce healthy cells! It is at this crucial stage of life woman can become more vulnerable to disease. This is our true connection to good nutrition, health and aging properly. Everything we put into our mouths, good or bad has a direct connection to our youthful body and how we feel at this stage of life. After my car accident, I decided to change my eating habits and replace my high protein, low carbohydrate diet with real food. My massage therapist, Leigh-lee told me of a diet that helped her lose 25 pounds in six months. It was in a book I knew long ago and remembered. The book was called *Fit for Life* by Dr. Edward Taub.

The book teaches you to group foods together and supply your missing vitamins and anti-oxidants in a timely manner. In the morning you have fruit juice (not concentrated) and fresh fruits, such as peaches, pears, berries and pineapples until noon. I truly thought that I would be starving, but actually I had more vitality and energy than ever before. You must drink plenty of water all day and after noon, you can have a variety of natural foods such as "energy salad" or two pieces of wheat bread slightly toasted and mixed with lettuce, tomato, cucumber, avocado, cauliflower and broccoli steamed. I mix up a mayonnaise/spicy mustard sauce and apply it to my toast and eat my sandwich. This would suffice until 3:00 p.m. Then I would either have more juice or more fresh vegetables until dinner. Dinner would consist of three to four ounces of protein, at least two to three vegetables and a salad if desired. I would eat steak only once a week, chicken or fresh fish was my favorite each night and I also ingested one glass of wine. This was not considered "healthy" on the Fit for Life diet, but I decided I would not give up my lifestyle completely.

This diet completely detoxifies your body and totally eliminates processed sugar, creating a more balanced insulin level. Imagine the insulin in your body looking unsuccessfully to store the abundance of glucose from all of the sugar we ingest, whether it is in the form of cakes, cookies or high starch vegetables or white flour and bread. Then just picture how the sugar gets converted into fat because your cells cannot accept anymore sugar. Just visualize these free radicals sweeping through your body and damaging your cells. It is not a pretty picture, but this is what happens and that is the main reason why older women cannot eat what they did when they were younger. Part of looking good and feeling good is in your internal health and combined with nutritious foods and exercise, we can help prevent the healthy cells from dying at a more rapid rate. When I feed my body properly, my cells thrive and I feel jubilant that I am fighting off disease and aging for as long as possible. Your healthy cells will keep you looking young, slim and feeling energetic again! We are going to age physically, but we have control over how we age and how well we age. Which individuals are in the best of health? It is no surprise, it is the ones who have exercised and eaten right for the last 20 years. Eating real foods, not processed foods, avoiding chemicals, exercising daily, drinking lots of water, getting plenty of rest, watching the consumption of alcohol and avoiding smoking all add up to looking great and feeling good! My personal trainer, Terry Walters always told me, you are what you eat and if you eat the processed foods, it goes right to your hips, shows in your skin tone and in your overall general health.

It takes more work and discipline than ever before to look good as you age, but you are the lucky one if you work hard at it. If you look around, it is easy to see who has given up. It happens to both men and women. First comes the weight gain and it continues to pile up if no thought is given to control it. Then after the weight gain has taken control, along comes the deteriorating bone loss and the general diseases will follow.

Most people think disease is part of aging and have no understanding of the ill effects of elevated insulin levels. Aging and disease go hand in hand. Bad lifestyles are the culprit of how we age. If you understand that you control your own health and have the power to change your own destiny, you then can make a devoted commitment to improve yourself. It's a choice, do I want to lie in bed or do I want to get up and walk or exercise or swim? Just get moving, whether it is cardiovascular training, weight training or yoga. Once you make this commitment, you will then start to watch your intake of food. Your sugar intake will lessen, your carbohydrates will diminish and you will lose more fat then you ever imagined!

Another important factor is caffeine. I love caffeine, but I have found through reading that caffeine blocks estrogen production, which eventually leads to insulin resistance and then to long term disease.

I have found green tea and decaffeinated coffee is not a bad alternative. One cup of java in the morning is good enough for me and for the rest of the day I drink decaffeinated coffee until the evening when I have a glass of red wine.... I know wine contains sugar, but I am not changing my lifestyle completely for the rest of my 50 years! If I feel this good, I may just live that long!

It is these changes that will set you on a path of heart and soul combined with good nutrition and excellent health. The choice is up to you and you will feel emotionally and physically happier!

NUTRITIONAL DIET

Our hormones and brains, indeed our entire physiology was designed to operate on the unadulterated whole foods that were available to the earliest humans. When we don't eat them we experience health problems: not only obesity, but reproductive problems, sexual dysfunction, PMS, migraines, and even cancer. By choosing foods that are compatible with your hormones, you can improve many of these conditions, and you will feel better while doing it!

This diet plan creates a hormone equilibrium that keeps you well balanced. It is designed to work with, rather than against, your old hormonal programming.

The Perfect Balance diet plan consists of plant foods and animal products-meat, fish, fowl, dairy, and eggs. Your daily intake is at least 75% plant food, and no more than 25% animal foods. Whole grains, fruits, vegetables, nuts and seeds, are rich in nutrients, low in calories, and full of antioxidants and phytoestrogens. If you follow the plan's principles-supplemented by plenty of water, antioxidant foods, and good fats-you'll be on the road to hormonal balance.

Power Carbs versus Chaos Carbs

Source	Power Carbs	Chaos Carbs
Grains	Barley; whole wheat such as wheat berries or cracked wheat; long grain wild rice; quinoa	Instant rice; short grain rice; white or refined flours
Breads	Oat-Bran; multigrain; whole-grain	White bread; white-flour bagels, rolls, baguettes
Legumes	Baked beans; chick peas; kidney bans; soybeans	Sweetened baked beans; peanut butter with hydrogenated oils; refried beans prepared with lard

Vegetables	Artichokes; asparagus; eggplant; all peppers; any dark-green leafy vegetables	French fries; instant potatoes; parsnips; beets
Fruit	Grapefruit; blueberries; cherries; plums	Canned Fruit cocktail; peaches in syrup; caramel apple; dried banana chips
Beverages	Skim milk; lowfat soy milk; tomato juice; hot cocoa	Soft drinks (non-diet); sports drinks, sweetened instant teas; whole milk latte
Sweets and Treats	Non-fat frozen yogurt; dark chocolate; low-fat granola	Whole-fat ice cram; doughnuts; packaged cookies; cheesecake

Perfect Foods

Source	Description
Oatmeal	Loaded with soluble and insoluble fiber, this Power Carb will stabilize your insulin levels while you gradually absorb the brain boosting sugars. Rich in fiber, oatmeal leaves your stomach slowly, suppressing your levels of a hormone called ghrelin, which in turn helps to shut off your appetite.
Eggs	These performance proteins promote the release of growth hormone and keep you alert throughout the morning. Choline is one of the macronutrients in eggs that gives your brain a much needed building block for one of your memory neurotransmitters, acetylcholine.
Nonfat Organic Milk	One cup gives you 9 grams of proteins without added toxins and synthetic growth hormones. It also provides 30 percent of you daily calcium to strengthen your bones and help you burn fats.

Soybeans	Loaded with cancer-fighting phytoestrogens, these protein powerhouses are the "thinking women's" best friend.
Organic Chili	A great insulin-stabilizing meal that includes beans for fiber and protein in the form of texturized vegetable protein or 90-95 percent organic lean ground beef. Chili suppresses your ghrelin levels, which keeps you feeling full longer.
Whole-Wheat Pasta	This Power Carb keeps insulin levels low but still supplies the flavor and texture to your favorite pasta. It is digested, and then released slowly as glucose when you need fuel for your muscles and brain.
Pomegranates	This exotic fruit contains a small amount of estradiol that will be absorbed slowly owing to the carbohydrates and proteins in the fruit. It will boost your own estrogen production and improve the way you feel.
Green tea	This drink fights free radicals with its anti-inflammatory and antioxidant properties. It also contains compounds thought to prevent certain cancers.
Red Wine	A glass before dinner will raise your testosterone level. This can give you that last bit of energy to get through the rest of the day while boosting your libido. Wine is also rich in antioxidants to protect your brain against free-radicals.
Dark Chocolate	This treat contains many antioxidants that protect your brain. It also has brain-boosting chemicals, including phenyl ethylamine (PEA), currently thought to be a primary neurotransmitter associates with passionate love.

ﾍ ﾍ ﾍ

Vitamins and Nutrients needed for Perimenopause and Menopause

- Vitamin C- 2000mg necessary a day for women

- Vitamin A- Helps with heavy bleeding during periods

- Vitamin B-12- Helps with mental function and depression

- Lecithin- May help with estrogen- based disorders such as uterine fibroids, endometriosis, and breast and fibrocystic breast syndrome.

- Inositol- Helps with depression, anxiety, and sleepless nights!

- Biotin- Can help with thinning of hair and help to improve general appearance of hair

- Vitamin C- Helps with stress and protects body from harmful toxins

- Ginkgo biloba- Brings oxygen and energy into the brain

- Grape Seed- Helps to curb heavy menstrual flows

- Vitamin D- Absorbs calcium better, and helps with your bone density

- Vitamin K- Helps with Osteoporosis and bone strength

- Calcium- Helps with bone loss, hypertension, high cholesterol, and Insomnia

- Magnesium- Helps with mood swings and also to tame premenstrual migraines and yeast infections. Also helps in better sleep!

- Iron- During the menstruating years, and needed when menopause begins (Must be checked by blood test to determine if low)

- Zinc- Sexual and reproductive health-a libido boost!

- Chromium- Excellent for heart disease, aging, diabetes, and can help chronic headaches

- Boron- Can help raise estrogen level, help with osteoporosis, and for women afraid of taking hormone therapy, also used to help with hot flashes.

- L-glutamine- Known to help sugar urges, tissue repair, and to help control cravings- even with alcohol addiction.

- Lysine- Helps prevent osteoporosis, keeps the heart strong and preserves muscle tissue

- Phenylalanine- Known as PA a neurotransmitter promotes alertness, positive disposition, and perhaps pain relief. Note: Physician supervision necessary, as can elevate blood pressure.

- GABA- For anxiety and depression during menstruation. Small doses are required, between 500mg - 4 grams daily.

- Carnitine- The fat burner, heart helper, and for energy and endurance, take between 500mg, or 1 gram for preventative purposes

- ALC- Helps to improve mood, mental energy, slows the aging of brain cells, and impede the advance of Alzheimer's. Take carnitine and ALC daily 500-1000mgs of both supplements together.

- Omega-3S- Fish oil for the heart, blood pressure, joint diseases, skin disorders, and mood disorders

- Flaxseed Oil- Helps with pre-menstrual tension- take fish oil and flaxseed oil together creating balance!

- GLA- PMS is helped best by this therapy, as well as breast tenderness and cramps- 300mgs daily dosage suggested , also promotes healthy skin!(known as Evening Primrose Oil, borage seeds, black currant seeds)

- Gamma-Oryzanol- Menopause hot flashes, night sweats diminish 30mgs- as much as 300 mgs, also digestive problems and helping to treat depression.

- DHEA- The mother hormone, improves sex drive, enhances immune function and keener memory. An antidote to help with aging!

- Pregnenolone- Sex steroid hormone makes it especially a vital supplement by creating a balance with estrogen to reduce the risk of certain cancers that develop in women. Also widely used in Atkins Center replacing the widely used prednisone. (Use under Dr. Orders)

- Melatonin- Best solution for insomnia, headaches, at the Atkins Center they use 12-20 mgs. For cancer patients having trouble with their sleeping. patterns. A dose between 1-3mgs nightly for a week helps acclimate you to a new sleep schedule.

- Ginkgo Biloba- Used mainly for PMS, but is wonderful for mental acuity, and headaches

- Bromelain- Used to relieve inflammation especially during chemical peels and face lift surgery

- Arnica- Also used during and after surgery to help relieve swelling and bruising

- St. John's Wort- Used as an antidepressant, and also helps to fight influenza

- Kava- Body and mind can relax with this herb, and can facilitate healing and pain relief.

- Valerian- Anxious? Try a few capsules of this herb before going to bed, and you can fall asleep without sleeping pills

- Cranberry- Known for helping urinary tract infection or recurrent bladder infections. (4-6 capsules) Juice contains too much sugar.

- Feverfew- Takes months, but helps in migraine therapy at Atkins Center

- Black cohosh- Use as extract for hot flashes or menopausal symptoms

- Calcium- You need at least 750-1500 mgs a day during menopausal times

- Wild Yam- Used as a topical progesterone cream for menopausal therapy, but not very effective

These therapies have been used at the Atkins Center and must be used carefully and some with Dr. Supervision necessary. Discuss these ideas with your Physician before implementing any vitamins or herbs, and more is not better!

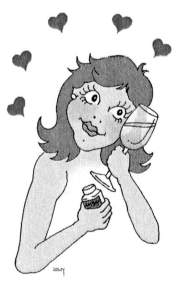

When Ambien and Chardonnay are your best friends!

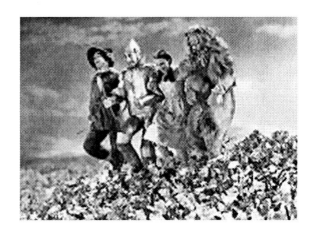

Chapter 14

Substance Abuse and Menopause: "Let's Not Help
Things Along"

By Linda LaVelle A.T.I.E. I.T.E.C.

When I asked the girls that work with me what they thought about what contributes to substance abuse, one of my massage therapists Suzie said: Men, Age, Sex, Children, and Money- all not in that order! After laughing I realized that she is definitely right, as all of these factors definitely contribute to the abuse of alcohol, the sleeping pills used to get a good night's sleep, or the pain killers to get you through the hard day of work? Some even abuse cocaine, marijuana, and heroin to cope with life's daily chores. This abuse gets even more accelerated when you add peri-menopause or menopausal factors to the picture.

When I first became perimenopausal, I seemed to be in search of my old self again, the one that wouldn't fly off the handle when asked a simple question, or go into a fit of depression and poor me blues during my weekly time. To add to this time, I had been praying for a child and to my blessings at 44 years of age, I had a baby boy! After delivering this beautiful bundle of joy, I quickly went into hormone ups and downs, and I knew nothing about this adventure! I can vividly remember stepping out on the patio to escape my screaming baby who needed me for his feeding, and I wanted to run away from the house just to escape his crying...I longed for peace and quiet, and I felt guilty that I was afraid to even hold him, much less feed him. I would walk him in his stroller and start crying for blocks as he would just sleep away in la la land. And I wondered if this was normal for these crying jags? I would wake up with night sweats and once I was done feeding the baby at 2a.m., I could not get back to sleep so I would take a Tylenol PM, and be literally knocked out until 7a.m. when my husband would hear the baby screaming and wonder why I didn't?

On weekends I would resort to drinking a bottle of Chardonnay Wine with occasional shots of Rum to ease my tensions from the new Mother Syndrome, and the new going back to work scene with all the stresses of daily life to boot! I was definitely in a tropical mood with Jimmy Buffett every weekend. This was my only way to relax and unwind, and I got no help from my husband at that time...he would just disappear to go play Golf, or go to work on the lawn and all of the plants that were in our yard. That seemed to be his escape from me and the baby, and I was in another world, and developing a Substance Abuse problem! By the time Monday morning rolled around, I was feeling bloated, headache, body ache and crabby as all Hell! I was in the blue doldrums, and where was Jimmy Buffett now when I really need him? I would stop on the way to work and hit McDonalds for a quick breakfast pick up laden with calories, a little java, and at lunch a cheeseburger with fries and a Coke... Oh, I was on my way all right, heading into a size 14 from a size 6, and I didn't much care what I looked like.

When I went for my monthly check up I was afraid to tell my gynecologist what was happening to me for fear that he would put me away and I would never see my baby again, but he was able to tell when he did a blood profile and asked me a few questions. I told him I had erratic behavior problems and that I had moody episodes and up and down moodiness. I also told him that I was having trouble sleeping at night, and that I had been depressed! I didn't want to tell him about the drinking binges or the Tylenol PM Etc, because I was truly embarrassed about my uncontrollable drinking and my inability to sleep at night. I truly thought that I was the only one that was going through this horrific time. When I finally told him about my erratic behavior and up and down moods, he suggested that I take Estrace during my monthly periods and I took more vitamin B complex as I heard that it was great for stress, and boy was I experiencing it! I also wanted to get back to a healthier approach to living through this bitchy up and down bloated, run yourself into a wall passage of life! I could see that it could get to a substance abuse situation and I was prepared to fight it all the way!

Now I was a typical perimenopausal woman going through the ups and downs of hormonal craziness, but never did I know or experience what was to come in the Menopause phase of life! This was like having perimenopause every day of your life, a revved up kind of version with no sense of normalcy in your every day kind of routine, it took over your body and would not let you go back to your old self as Peri-menopause would give you a break for 2-3 weeks, this is unrelenting and continues on till you want to scream for help!!!

I started my diet again to try and get my self back to 140 lbs again, and with a trainer on my butt I finally after 3 months was starting to see my old self coming back to life again! I lost 25 lbs and I was working out 3-4 days a week doing weight lifting and cardio, a total of ½ hour for each activity, and watching my calorie intake of food as well as my intake of alcohol. I found that by nighttime, I was really exhausted from the workout as well as the day's activities, and I did not need to take any pill to put me to sleep! I was doing absolutely great for 3-4 years and maintaining my weight and sanity until menopause finally hit me around the age of 49 years...

The periods were getting more frequent, 2 weeks apart to be exact. The moods were getting crazier and I was going into high anxiety combined with moments of calmness. Then came the heart palpitations and missed heart beats. I was really trying to be as calm as possible, but what was up with this rapid heart beat and rise in blood pressure? I now thought I was literally going nuts, and I was told to go and see a Cardiologist to see what was up with this passage in life!

He wanted to put me through a series of tests, and the stress test he never asked me to perform, because he and I would spend close to ½ hour on the treadmill next to each other and talk through the whole working episode, so I figured that he thought it might be my genetic background as I was beginning to think that as well. My father died at 46 years of age of a heart attack and we had no clue if he had high blood pressure or if he had high cholesterol problems because in the 1960's there were no reports out about the repercussions of heart problems or what to do to help yourself. You just died and you went on with life. When my mother died at 70 years of heart problems sustained with alcohol abuse, I knew that I had to watch myself for the rest of my life if I was to live longer than 70 years of age, and with a baby boy in my arms I set out to find the best way to keep my health in check! I just was not prepared with Menopause and what you experience with this wonderful passage!

Now getting back to my Cardiologist. He suggested that I have a Holter Monitor placed on my body for a period of 24 hours to see if I was having heart palpitations and high anxiety problems. You see, I don't think anyone believed that I was actually going through this. They knew my blood pressure was high, but couldn't find a cardiovascular problem. They literally brushed it off to anxiety attacks. You cannot live on these pills every day of your life as you will miss ½ of the days adventures and fits of craziness that occur with your every mundane life! After getting rid of the Holter Monitor test they found that my heart was skipping a beat now and then, and yes they finally believed that I was not crazy. These symptoms that I was experiencing were for real… Heart palpitations and high blood pressure (combined with a few anxiety attacks thrown in).

I was now looking for a peaceful more relaxed life. My cardiologist suggested Lorezapem for the anxiety attacks and Inderal for the erratic heartbeats that were occurring. I could see that you could really get caught up in all these medications, and I wanted to be free of them completely, so I set out again to find out the real cause of these problems. Just guess what the main problem was?

Menopause!!! My hormones were not properly regulated as I was trying the natural approach to this passage of life, a little of estroven, black cohosh, a lot of Soy milk and Calcium for the bones. It was definitely not working, I hated everyone including myself, and my hot flashes were about 25 a day, as well as night sweats every 3-4 hours. I was the bitchy bloated working out wonder with a great body and no calmness of mind or spirit! No wonder I was turning to drugs and alcohol to ease my soul!

Every 6 months, my internist would ask for a blood count as well as a urine specimen in my meeting with him. Each time that he would see me, he told me that he found a trace of blood in my urine. I then set out on a mission to find out if there was anything wrong with my bladder or kidneys, etc. I went to a urologist, and he sent me on a myriad of tests from a proctology exam that you should have at age 50 years, to a kidney test, MRI test of the bladder and kidneys, and CT scans of every part of my body. The urologist told me after all the tests were negative, just don't worry about it, this problem is not life threatening and he would see me in another year. By the way, he said that I had the prettiest bladder he had ever seen!

That was a year ago, and I still have the blood in my urine after a recent blood test, but I guess we have to have something wrong with our bodies. We are actually a century year old and things will go wrong from now on, so get used to this way of life!

I am telling you this so that you realize that strange things happen during the menopausal years, and I want you to learn as much as you can to counteract these strange occurrences during this passage of life!

Let us get back to substance abuse, and why we let this happens. It is very easy to get caught up in alcohol, drugs, cocaine, marijuana, and prescription drug abuse. You are definitely not in your right frame of mind during menopause, and combined with an outer body experience happening. I can well understand the explosion of substance abuse. I have been very fortunate to have a good psychotherapist to help me get through this passage of life. Now if any one had the right to get involved with substance abuse, it certainly was me, and looking back at this passage of time I can see why it would occur with me. Looking back at my past 10 years I had some devastating losses.

During the last few years from 47- 53 years of age, I went through a divorce, I lost my mother, I lost my Brother, I lost 3 Shih-Tzu dogs, I went from a 4,000 square foot house on the river to a 1,600 square foot small cramped house with my son, and I was forced into the single life again! By age 50, I finally met a man that wanted to share my life with my son and me, and we made our move back into a beautiful house again and got married and he adopted my son Sean. Now everything was going along smooth until menopause set in, and more strange medical problems cropped up!

My Aunt who was just like my mother passed on, and I was left with the problems of taking care of an elderly uncle that was in need of nursing care and full- time care with a limited budget! I guess due to the stress of so much placed on my plate you think that I would start drinking or take pills, but before I could even think of that along comes "Double Vertigo" a condition that leaves you perfectly helpless, crawling on the floor for help, and virtually throwing up if you try to stand up. You end up just falling into bed praying that the room around you will stop spinning in circles. Just to have your balance again is a prayer I prayed for weeks. I still to this day do not know why this occurred, and the doctor seems to think that it was stress induced, but it did cause injury to my right ear where there is 40% nerve damage. I had to learn to walk and move my head with balance lessons and train my eyes to see balance correctly. It took about 6 months of hard work and recuperation along with taking Valium to help ease my dizzy spells. They gradually dissipated, and I set out to find out why this horrible event really occurred. My Ear Nose and Throat Doctor seems to think that there was a sudden change in my blood pressure either low or high, but that it definitely was pressure related causing me to have the sudden drop in my blood pressure was devastating to my body resulting in the double Vertigo problem. All of this during the Menopausal stage of life! I actually was afraid to try and stop taking my Valium pills for fear that my vertigo would come knocking at my door again. I was feeling like my old self again; I just kept taking them nightly without realizing that they were addicting.

When I went to my gynecologist and told him that I was having trouble sleeping, he asked what I was taking for night time sleep. When I told him that I was taking valium, he calmly told me that besides being addicting, they help you to lose your memory. Well that was all I needed to change that bad habit. I always thought that the "Dumb Blonde" was a joke but the idea of losing my memory was no laughing matter. It was happening and I was excusing it as a part of menopause. I was forgetting to go to the bank, or the dry cleaners etc. All the programmed things that you normally do were being thrown off kilter with this pill I was taking! I decided to kick the habit of Valium, and my doctor gave me some samples of Ambien to try and have good nights sleep. I tried Ambien and it finally put me into REM sleep! I felt like a new woman again, and believe me; you will do just about anything to have one good night of sleep. I can see why you can also get addicted to Ambien, and it is no wonder why so many women are hooked on Tylenol PM or Ambien. I have decided that I will only take Ambien when I am restless and waking up between 10pm and 12pm, as I don't want to fall prey to another addiction to any drug.

The wonderful news is that my gynecologist found a Mirena IUD that allows my progesterone to stay in my uterus helping that area with the hormone I was missing, and I sleep great at night now, without the help of any drugs! It is very important to get your hormones in proper check during this passage, and surprisingly things fall back in place. I still have blood pressure problems, I still have blood in my urine, but I am well balanced in my thoughts of everyday life, and my memory is back as strong as it used to be before all the craziness!

Now I hope that you can see how Substance Abuse can easily get started, and it is up to you to prevent it from happening. The Medical Doctors are here to help guide us through this passage, but it is up to you to take full control of your mind, soul, and body to prevent abuse from developing into a serious issue. We all have an inner guidance system, the soul to some, the psyche to others, and it is always speaking to us moving us in the right direction. You must learn to pay attention to what it says and follow its lead in the right path. I now see that in the second half of my life I have a new journey to accomplish, Self Discovery without Self Abuse.

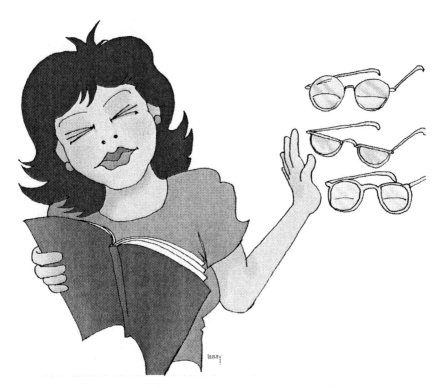

When you need 3 pairs of eye glasses to function,
and you really don't want to put them on!

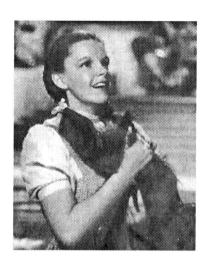

Chapter 15

Facelifts & Chemical Peels

By Stephen C. Adler, M.D. and Linda LaVelle

History

The search for beauty and lasting youth has intrigued many throughout the ages. During the Classical Period in Greece (428-348 BC) Plato studied proportions of the body that defined beauty, and even prizes were awarded for beauty. Statues of figures like Aphrodite and Venus de Milo represented ideal proportions of face and body and defined beauty for centuries. The Renaissance Period from the late 14th century to the mid 16th century provided a blending of science, architecture, art, humanism and philosophy which transcended previous definitions of ideal beauty for both male and female figures. Leonardo DaVinci studied the ideal proportions of the human body in his work of the Vitruvian Man (circa 1480), and ideal beauty characteristics were presented by the most admired painting Mona Lisa (1503-1506). Michelangelo Bounarti in his study of the ideal man, sculpted the David (1501-15030), which represented strength and beauty of the

Renaissance man. Raphael of Urbino (Madonna of the Grand Duke) and Sandro Boticelli (Primavera and Birth of Venus) presented beauty form the physical to the expressive nature of their works. In the 15th century, Ponce de Leon was searching for the fountain of youth during his travels in the New World. From the 17th century to the present times beauty was portrayed from physical beauty to elaborate garments and fashion. Hair styles, jewelry, cosmetics, makeup, anti-aging, weight loss, physical fitness, and dental aesthetics provide a multitude of options contributing to achieve ideal beauty.

Plastic surgery has revolutionized and evolved in the last 100 years to help achieve and preserve the ideals of beauty. Facelift surgery has been performed since the early 1900's by German and French surgeons. Dr. Lexer(1906), Dr. Hollander(1912), Dr. Joseph (1921) and Dr. Passot (1919) were among the first to perform aging face surgery.

The early facelifts just provided a purely skin lift which resulted in a short term result and when pulled excessively provided an unnatural and pulled appearance. The advanced facelift techniques evolved in the 1970's which involved pulling muscle and skin in order to achieve a long lasting and natural result.

Before discussing the technical and recovery aspects of facelifts and chemical peels, I will share my personal philosophy regarding the evolution and the goals of our work.

Personal Philosophy

The face is the most important feature of the body, and it represents a social passport to society. Unlike other body areas which can be easily camouflaged or hidden with wardrobes and covers, the face is open and visible.

The face must look natural to look beautiful; the face must look natural to look youthful. The exaggerated and altered appearance seen in some patients who have undergone aggressive facelifts is not attractive, but disturbing. As surgeons, we must evaluate and re-evaluate our results to assure that our patients follow our philosophical view of our work.

I see myself as a surgeon who tries to mimic nature, who strives to maintain the natural appearance and balance of the face. The greatest fear of patients is that they are afraid they will look different or like someone else after facial surgery. The fear of looking altered is real, the fear is often fueled by the tabloids and magazines which show movie stars and entertainers with disturbing appearances resulting from plastic surgery. As a surgeon, I keep patients looking like themselves. I appreciate the variability between different faces and their contours, contours that have to be softened and enhanced, and not removed or distorted. I see myself as a surgeon who examines the faces in great detail, but promotes doing the least to get the most of results.

I had the experience where I saw a patient in consultation having previous facial surgery before coming to see me. She was unhappy because of her altered and pulled appearance. I tried to guess her age, which is something I rarely do. I guessed her to be in her early 60's. I looked at the chart, and found that she was only 52 years of age. It was then that I realized that pulling more does not make people look younger, better or more attractive.

Patients often come complaining of heavy jowls, nasal folds and loose neck. They often think that it all has to be pulled completely to get the desired results. I disagree, and I discuss with them that if you pull the neck completely tight, completely remove the jowls and flatten the marionette area, and completely remove the nasal folds they will look like they are in an open cockpit of an airplane.

When you look at that woman who obviously had overdone plastic surgery (usually walking in the mall), ask several questions? Is her neck tight- yes, are her jowls completely gone-yes, are her nasal folds flat and removed-yes, are the lines on the face completely gone-yes, does she look better-NO, does she look natural-NO, does she look attractive-NO, does she look younger-NO. She obviously looks altered and operated, she does not look young or attractive. She looks like an old lady with a bad facelift. It is ok to have folds, it is ok to have contours on the face (even babies do!), hey it is even ok to have some lines on the face.

My goal, just like the artist of the Renaissance Period, is to strive to achieve a natural result, one where balance and symmetry are maintained, one which looks more beautiful and attractive. I believe you can be beautiful and attractive in your 30's, 40's, 50's, 60's, 70's, and above, only and only if you look natural. Patients undergoing plastic surgery of the face should not look like they had plastic surgery.

Facelift

The facelift operation is a procedure that accomplishes several objectives. The objective is to remove excess skin, tighten loose muscle and in some cases remove unwanted fat through the combination of liposuction on the neck and jawline.

Consultation

It is important that the physician and patient have good communication and understanding of the problems and the possible solutions. It is important to have written information for the patient so that they may be better informed on the procedure and recovery. Patient need to understand that facelift does, and what it does not do. Facelifts do not remove wrinkles, it removes sagging skin and folds. Chemical peels and laser resurfacing improves lines and wrinkles.

During the consultation patients understands how aging is related to heredity, and at the same time get educated about the procedure. Patients often comment on how they are looking like their parents.

During the consultation, the patients will learn about aging, loss of elasticity, gravity, and loss of soft tissue or volume. Review of social history can reveal problems such as smoking, sun exposure, stress, hormonal changes and how these contribute to premature aging. Review of medical history may reveal problems like diabetes, hypertension, heart or lung diseases and any other medical problems that must be identified and controlled prior to surgery. I always require a full medical work-up and clearance from an internist or family physician, laboratories to check blood chemistries, coagulation and hemoglobin and EKG-electrocardiogram. My goal is to produce the safest environment and achieve the best aesthetic results.

A physical exam in front of a mirror allows for a thorough evaluation. I like to feel the soft tissue on the face and palpate the relaxation, elasticity and folding of the tissues in the cheek, jowl and neck. I also like to examine other areas such as prejowl area, marionette line, chin projection and lips, which may require combined procedures such as fillers, fat transfers, chin-prejowl implant or lip enhancement procedures.

I discuss anesthesia, the healing process, and what to expect at different stages in the post operative period. I stress the importance that changes will happen from several weeks to several months after surgery. I also discuss the risks, limitations, possibility of additional treatments and/or medical measures, and factors associated with wound healing.

Computer imaging can be used to enhance the consultation. This tool can be used to show the patient what can be accomplished with the surgery, as well as the limitations. The computer imaging is not a guarantee of results and this must be conveyed to the patient to avoid unrealistic expectations.

Educating the patient and evaluation of physical and emotional expectations is my goal during the consultation. I believe that well informed patients can make better decisions. I also encourage second consultations because of the information overload during the initial visit. Patient may have questions after the initial visit.

Medications to avoid prior to surgery encompass a wide array of aspirin, and all aspirin-like substances. Ibuprofen, Motrin, Advil, anti-inflammatories among many others. Make sure you review all medications with your doctor, be give a list of medications to avoid.

Herbs, natural supplements must also be avoided because of possible interference with anesthesia and clotting. Vitamins must also be avoided, like Vitamin E.

Procedure

The incision planning and placement are of crucial importance to hide these facial scars. The hairline has to be considered and preserved so that it is not altered. Altered hairlines are a sign of an unnatural facelift because the face looks bigger for the size of the head. Avoiding the pulled earlobe look also preserves the natural look.

The operation accomplishes the pulling of skin, tightening of muscle and removing unwanted fat. The operation may take an average of two to four hours, and can be performed with other procedures such as: endoscopic browlifts, eyelid surgery, fat transfers, lip procedures, and skin resurfacing.

Recovery

After the surgery the patient wears head dressing which stays overnight and is removed the next morning. The patient sleeps with the head elevated at least 30 degrees, and receives cold compresses throughout the first week. I find cold compresses help reduce swelling and discomfort. Swelling peaks at three days and 80% is gone in 2 weeks, 90% in two months and the last 10% go at a rate of 1% per month for the next year. Bruising is variable, but most is gone between

7-14 days. Pain is usually mild to moderate, and responds to mild narcotic analgesics. Many patients just take Tylenol® after the first 2-3 days. Sleeping medication is used only when needed. The incision lines are cleaned multiple times daily, and coated with antibiotic ointment.

Patients may go through an emotional rollercoaster during the first few weeks. After the surgery there is a feeling of elation and excitement, then within several days there could be a feeling of depression. Emotional support is of importance during this time.

Sutures are removed at one week, and most patients can resume normal social activities at about 2 weeks. Of course, there is still much to change even after 2 weeks. During the post operative period patients need to be reassured as needed.

Exercise and heavy activities such as weight lifting, golf, tennis and swimming must be put on hold for 4 weeks. Light leisure walking can be started at one week, and more active strenuous walking at about 3 weeks.

Chemical Peels and Skin Resurfacing

The treatment of facial wrinkles continues to challenge physicians and surgeons. The desire to have youthful and attractive skin has been present for centuries. Cleopatra use milk baths, which contained high levels of lactic acid (B-hydroxy acid) to maintain a youthful and beautiful skin. The early 80's revolutionized the skin care industry with the introduction of glycolic acids which acted as strong moisturizers and exfoliants.

Billions of dollars are spent each year on cosmetics, sun protection products and other prescription lotions such as Retin A, alpha hydroxyl acids and others to attain smoother and more attractive skin.

Medical treatment of wrinkles has evolved from chemical treatments and recently with the use of lasers.

It is important to understand that we, as physicians, must look at new technology critically, and accept it only when results are corroborated by scientific data and research.

We must not forget that older treatments are effective and have passed the test of time in proving their safety and results. Newer is not always better in plastic surgery.

How does a peel or laser work? The principle mechanism in all forms of peel and laser is to remove old, superficial, pigmented, and wrinkled skin and replace it with newly formed, tighter, smoother and younger appearing skin. The "new" skin contains new collagen, and elastic fibers which are produced by the deeper layers of the skin.

How is the layer removed? We can use chemical peels, dermabrasion and lasers. Most important is to understand the different levels of the skin which are treated in different resurfacing techniques. The principles of peels applied are that skin can be removed in different levels, superficial, intermediate and deep. Depending on how deep the peel penetrates, the difference in results and recovery. The deeper the peel the more improvement, but also more the recovery and risks associated with the treatment.

What is the difference between Microdermabrasion and Dermabrasion? Microdermabrasion is a light superficial treatment performed by aestheticians to improve the texture of the skin and remove mild discoloration. Dermabrasion is a deep peel performed by a physician using a wire or diamond burr that mechanically removes the surface of the skin in order to improve acne scars, wrinkles, irregular and uneven skin. These treatments must not be confused since they are utilized for totally different problems.

Superficial Chemical Peels

Superficial chemical peels are also referred as to "lunch time" or "complexion" peels. These are performed in the office, with glycolic acid 15%, 30% or 50%. These peels promote softer and smoother skin, treat minor pigment changes and sun damage with minimal effect on wrinkles. They are usually performed in a series to get the most benefit from the sequential exfoliation. These can be performed several times a year, and can help diminish the signs of aging skin.

How are these performed?

The face is cleaned and dried with alcohol or even acetone. This step is performed to remove the fatty oils from the skin, which allows the glycolic acid to penetrate evenly. The chemical is applied to skin with a cotton ball, and cotton tip applicators for eyelid areas. After 3-5 minutes, the chemical peel is neutralized with a bicarbonate neutralizer or water rinses. A light moisturizer is applied prior to the patient's departure, and patient may return to work or the usual daily activities. Sun protection is important following any chemical treatment of the skin.

There is minimal stinging during these chemical peels, the skin may become reddish after the peel, and after several days there might be a flakiness associated with this exfoliation.

Intermediate Chemical Peel

This is the workhorse of all peels. These are known as the "mask" peels. The intermediate peel is very versatile, in that it addresses many different problems in the skin. It is a truly resurfacing peel which improves texture, surface, spots, wrinkles, discoloration and even some superficial skin cancers.

The chemicals used are Trichloroacetic Acid 25-35% (TCA) and is used in combination with Jessner's formula (Salicylic Acid 14% and Lactic Acid 14%). The skin is cleaned with alcohol or acetone to degrease the skin. Jessner's solution is applied and after 10 minutes the same is repeated with TCA 25% or 35%. The skin turns white like snow, and this represents the coagulation of proteins in the skin. The skin within minutes turns pink, and then the skin becomes taut and brownish. The skin looks like a mask, and within 3-5 days, it starts to peel like. After the peeling is complete, the skin is slightly pink, and people can resume their activities, and of course plenty of sunblock.

The intermediate peel is one of my favorite skin treatments because it provides a wide array of improvement with relatively less recovery than the deep peels.

Deep Peels

Deep peels can be classified as CO2 Laser, Phenol, or Dermabrasion. The importance of deep peels is that they all penetrate to approximately the same level in the skin. The deep peels result in a raw appearance of the skin, which takes approximately 7-10 days to form the new skin. Deep peels improve texture, resurface the skin, remove spots, sun damage, remove wrinkles, tighten the skin, and can even remove some superficial skin cancers. These peels require at least 1-2 week recovery, sun avoidance for 4-6 weeks, and without doubt, sun block 60-65 SPF.

Patients must understand that redness is a normal effect and part of the recovery. Redness may last from 3-4 weeks to several months. Eventually all redness dissipates, and patients must take care of their skin like a baby's skin. It is also important to select patients for deep peels, especially because some type III skin and darker skin types are not candidates for deep peels. Peels can cause discoloration and lightening of the skin in dark skinned individuals.

Risks of all peels range from hyperpigmentation, discoloration, prolonged redness, hyperpigmentation and scars.

Face Lifts and Chemical Peels

Embarking on facial plastic surgery or chemical peels is a significant step. Nobody makes the decision lightly. That is why Dr. Stephen Adler has dedicated himself to providing the utmost in comfort to his patients. His work ranges from facelifts to endoscopic browlifts, from chin and cheek implants to facial liposuction, and chemical peels to botox and restylane fillers. He is a true compassionate conservative, and seeks the least invasive means of delivering natural beauty to his patients. I was fortunate to have received the results of natural looking beauty, and it has changed my life forever! Dr. Adler is located in Stuart, Florida and has many board certifications.

I will now tell you my personal story about my Face Lift and Chemical Peel experience, and maybe this story will help you to make up your own mind and motivate you to trying surgery or just having a chemical peel to improve your skin.

I can vividly remember my 47th birthday. I went on a beautiful Disney Cruise with my so called wonderful husband of 7 years! We took our little son Sean who at the time was 3 years of age. As you know, I had this beautiful jewel at 44 years of age and was trying to avoid menopause like the plague! It was really working and I was still looking really good until my husband of 7 years announced on my Anniversary and Birthday Cruise that I was too old for him, my blonde hair was not brunette (no fooling!) and I did not excite him any more, as well as I was too old for him, and he wanted a divorce!!

The first thing I did was to find out where my son was on the cruise, and luckily he was in Adventure Ocean having a blast, and we were having a "romantic dinner" in a beautiful Italian Restaurant that you actually could create a beautiful child after this dinner and after dinner drinks! I of course succumbed to a husband that was very unhappy with everything I was! After the dinner and drinks, I checked in to Adventure Ocean brought Sean back to my room and put him to bed. My husband went out to a party for "singles" and I ordered a bottle of wine and sat out on the veranda and proceeded to drink the whole bottle of wine. I was on a ship headed for no where and my marriage was headed for the same course. I went in to take a shower and realized that my whole dream of a happy marriage and a beautiful life was quickly fading as well as a body that was quickly going south. I looked at my face after a night of crying, and boy did I look old! I made my mind up that as soon as I got home to Florida I was going to look up a Plastic Surgeon to fix my sagging breasts, and then I will go to my close friend Dr. Stephen Adler and see what he can do for my face?! I was excited but definitely scared of being single again. At 47 years of age, I did not want to be out dating and looking for Mr. Right! I thought that I had carefully researched this life long dream... After all, I had lost a husband at 39 years of age to a heart attack, and I was never going there again so I wanted a sperm specimen that would be a great catch for anyone that was dreaming of a perfect child, and I had certainly found it in my second husband! Boy was I wrong…and now I am looking at Breast Implants and Eye Tucks as well as a Chemical Peel to erase all the age spots from years of sun and fun!

When I got home from that fateful trip, I got a divorce within 3 months and within 6 months I was visiting Dr. Hilton Becker in Palm Beach Fla. and looking for a complete makeover. He suggested that I get breast implants for my saggy breasts and that I get an eye tuck and Chemical Peel to enhance my "New You". I got the breasts completed, and that was put on a Visa Card which I gladly paid for 3 years. My eyes waited for a few years, as I was busy raising Sean working on my own with a Spa Business and trying to make everyone else look beautiful!

The Plastic Surgeon in Stuart, Fla that I had been sending my clients to for several years was Dr. Stephen Adler, and his work was exemplary! He was truly an artist at creating the face that you were 10 years previous, and I visited him with a vision that I would look 10 years younger than my age. He looked at my sagging chin, my sagging eyes, and said "I will always keep you looking young". I believed him with my heart and soul, and proceeded to schedule a eye tuck with a chemical peel as well as a mini-lift to take away that awful chin that you see in pictures. That was disgusting and now I knew why my husband went for a younger girl! I was turning into the housefrau that everyone talks about!

I never realized what this all encompassed as all surgeons say that you are young and will get over it quickly! Quickly is not what happened as I want tomorrow to happen in an instant, and hello..I have to work for a living, so let's get on with this surgery and recover quickly! Well, things don't work that way, and the pain from the surgery was not so bad. I definitely looked like I was in a bar room brawl and lost! The pain was alleviated by Tylenol with Codeine, and I used 2 herbal remedies to alleviate the swelling and bruising. The glazed look on the first day was easy to handle, and I was enveloped in Vaseline and antibiotics and plenty of ice. By the second day, my nerve endings are going crazy with pain. The cold compresses are not helping, and I am allergic to codeine and swelling up like a balloon! My redness is extreme as I have Rosacea and now I am looking at my swollen face wondering what in the hell I have done to create this swollen blob looking at me? The first 3days I thought were scary, but the next two days were really eye opening! The skin was starting to peel and I didn't want to wait until I went to the doctor's office, so I slowly peeled off the dead cells that were lying on the top of my skin. I nearly fainted from the sight of this peeling procedure! I am a Skin Care Specialist and I truly thought that I could handle this peeling, but when it is your own dead skin it is different, and the pain in certain areas is excruciating especially around the nose and lip area. This occurred around the 5th day. It is very sensitive to air, and I used more Vaseline and witch hazel to cool it down. Many cool compresses were applied, you lie down for a few minutes and allow the skin to absorb the cold compresses, and then you go and attack the dead skin that is lying around waiting to be stripped from the skin. It is a Skin Care Technician's life long dream to rip the dead skin off of your face, but it is not the dream to rip your own skin off.

My 6th and 7th days were spent doing the cold compresses and using lip gloss to alleviate the dryness on my lips. I thought that if I would use my own products and my gentle masques, I would be in better shape. Boy was I ever wrong. Everything was super sensitive and I was getting redder and more Rosacea was developing on my raw skin. I just kept taking Tylenol for pain and applying cold compresses to alleviate the pain and swelling. Normally, the pain pills that they give you would help, but I was allergic to Codeine, so I had only Tylenol to deal with and ice packs so it is just punishment for my choosing to change my face. Believe me, when I get anything done to better myself, I look at it as just punishment to better myself, and I put up with the pain for how ever long it lasts, as it is worse to keep looking at your self with sagging eyes, downward chin and folds of skin under your chin, as well as age spots and wrinkles accumulating around the eye area.

On the eigth day, I was finally able to use my own products, and it was wonderful. I sprayed my toner on to my skin; I applied my vita plus masque to my face, and removed the rest of my dead cells from my skin. I then applied Vaseline to my skin, and went to bed. I was seeing Dr. Adler in the morning. The stitches still hurt around my ear area and I still felt very tight, but I knew it was only a matter of days before I would have my comfortable skin back again.

When I visited him he took the stitches out of my ear area and my eye area and said that I healed very quickly. I really think that they tell you this so that you feel very superb considering you looked like a swollen jelly fish. You really don't care however, you just want to go and shop and buy new cosmetics for your new found skin and face!

I had the perfect place to go-my own Salon. However, I couldn't use my own products for 2 weeks! I had the most sensitive products ever and could not touch them until Dr. Adler said that I was well again. I felt like a little girl without makeup, and I didn't want to go out and see anyone looking at my face red as it was and swollen like a melon! On the 10th day, I had to go to work, and I put on as much makeup as I could and went in to work with a very swollen face. The skin looked glazed and without wrinkles so I really didn't care what people thought. I felt 10 years younger and people really thought that I had had a really restful sleep the night before! Little did they know that I had been through 10 days of face lift makeover! Whatever, it was really worth it, whether it last 10 years like they predict or 15 years, it really doesn't matter because your face has taken 10 years south and you feel much younger! I can't say enough about the expertise and the artistry that Dr. Adler performed on my face. He gave me my self confidence back, and everyone that I met said how wonderful and relaxed I looked!

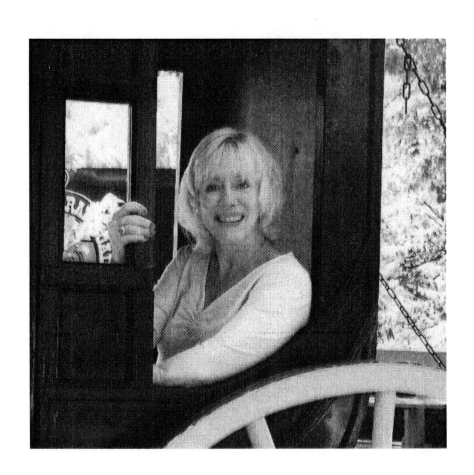

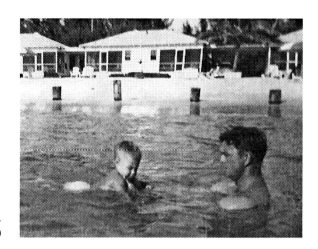

Chapter 16

For Men Only!

By Linda LaVelle A.T.I.E. I.T.E.C.

This chapter is specifically meant for the man who is living with his significant other in her passage of menopause! Just imagine for one moment that your Johnson, piggly wiggly, penis, etc has lost all of its power and hormones. It is completely dead, and has absolutely no hormones pumping through your shaft of life. Well, that is what a woman experiences when she enters Menopause. Now when you have male problems, you would experience about 3-4 problems that can get solved by a medical prescription or a hormone replacement. A woman has about 25 things that can go wrong with her, and it is up to her physician to put the puzzles and pieces together, wrap it up in 3 hormones estrogen, progesterone, and testosterone, and give them the right doses and make all 25 symptoms disappear. It is not as easy as it looks, and it sometimes takes years to figure the right replacement out for each woman's body...That is why patience and understanding comes in to play at this time.

How would you like to have hot flashes all day at work? First you are hot then you are cold, with night sweats where you would rip off your underwear and then put it back on within 10 minutes? Better yet, tell someone off just for the hell of it, go into your office and wonder where that outburst came from and better yet, what are you in your office for? Now, try and keep your household running efficiently handling all of the family's chores and dealing with craziness and memory loss. This is not an easy thing to do, and post it notes are laden everywhere for help. Your once happy disposition now becomes very moody and down right bitchy. You don't desire sex because you're Johnson has no testosterone pumping into it, and your once svelte figure is now gaining weight rapidly, and a big pot belly is emerging. Your hair which was once full and dark is now changing to thin and balding as well as silver in color. Your once happy eyes are drooping, and the color is not so bright anymore, much less you can't see as well because old age is setting in, and you can't see close up or far for that matter! Your feet hurt from retained water in your legs, and your mind is in an outer body experience looking for a good night's sleep like you used to have. You now get up at 2a.m. and cannot fall fast asleep anymore. You are thinking of a million things that can go wrong with the next day, and your partner is sound asleep next to you.

These are just some of the things that Menopausal women suffer from, your better half that you have loved for a few years or a half a century; it doesn't matter because this passage of life must have extreme patience and love behind it. We are temporarily lost souls searching for our safe return to our bodies, and with your love and understanding we can get back!

Please men, just put your baseball hats on when it is too cold, put your socks on your feet when you go to bed and if it is too cold, keep your mouth closed and bite your tongue when you want to call us stupid or forgetful. When we get up at 2 A.M., just give us a hug and an understanding nod and let us get up and do our thing. Please don't rag on us that we woke you up, and that you can't sleep because we know that you will be snoring within minutes and we will be sitting looking out the window trying anything to be where you are, in the middle of REM sleep! When we lack our sexual desire, I know it is hard for you to consider this, but get some candles burning, put some nice mood music on to calm our mind, and get us so excited right where we need it! Now that is a great start, and for most women just your understanding and love will put them in the sexy mood that you are in!

If our hot flashes kick in and we are in the middle of dinner, stop watching your show and go over and help your significant other. If the night sweats come on, turn the fan up so we can sweat easier, and remove the covers for us, so we can take our damn clothes off quickly. When we want to put our head in the freezer, open the refrigerator door and let us stay in there for a minute or two. I got a new refrigerator because it did have a gigantic freezer and I didn't mind spending the extra money for the convenience of that big compartment. At the time of purchase, my husband wondered why I wanted that large freezer. If he knew at the time that it was for my head, we never would have traded in our old fridge.

No one said that this passage of life would be easy, but you will have a happy and contented partner and a more loving woman if you can just understand a little how menopause really works. I really think that the divorce rate would definitely lessen if men and women had a better understanding of Menopausal Issues that occur during this time of life. I wish that a simple pill could solve all of our problems, but as you know this is a dream and you just have to look at us as a Work In Progress.

Always remember that behind every successful man there is and understanding woman pushing you to be your best. Washing your clothes, picking up your underwear, making your dinner, going to the store for your supplies, and giving you sex as much as she can. Listen Men, we put up with all of your embellishments (bad moods, farts, spits, blowing out your nostrils in the shower, belches, and loud snoring and bad breath) just to name a few of these wonderful traits. Please try and give us the love and understanding and peace that we so longingly deserve. One day a year is devoted to Mothers Day, and really that is just not enough. Just give us 10 minutes of your valuable time every evening, listen to our woes and complaints and we will love you forever!

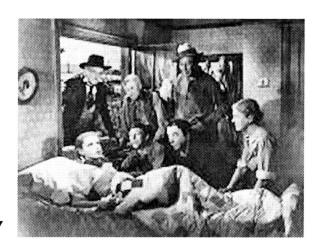

Chapter 17

Final Thoughts and Epilogue Four Years Post WHI Study: What Have We Learned and Where Do We Go From Here?

By Neil C. Boland, M.D., F.A.C.O.G. and Linda Lavelle, I.T.E.C., A.T.I.E.

Here in late 2006, we stand much more knowledgeably educated than we did in 2002 about menopause and how we can more safely help patients improve their quality of life. We are indeed now somewhere "over the rainbow" and Dorothy and little dog Toto have come back home again to be with Auntee Em. Glenda the Good Witch of Hormonal Therapy (GWHT) is triumphant again. The Wicked Witch of Evil Hormonal Therapy (WWEHT) however, now is now wounded instead of Glenda. We have visited Oz, and most of us have discovered we really did not like it there. Severe menopausal symptoms can be horrendous and deleterious to women's quality of life. We have awakened from our bad dream. ***There's no place like home........***

Hormonal therapy is now officially back in vogue, and the pendulum is now swinging back in favor of HT among the cognoscenti of the academic world. It's been discovered that when we look even more carefully at the WHI, there is so much more than "hormonal therapy is dangerous". It probably is dangerous if we select the wrong patient to prescribe it for. However, we have rediscovered that HT, properly prescribed for the right patient is not only rejuvenating, but is integrally important for high quality of life. Careful and deliberate weighing of HT benefits and risks for each individual patient is of paramount importance. As your health care provider, we carry a huge burden in continuing to monitor this benefit/ risk ratio as you age. Most women truly want to slow down the aging process, and not look and feel old before their time.

I heartily commend and congratulate the Womens Health Initiative Group of investigators for a first class long term study of the multiple dimensions of hormonal therapy and its impact on our patient's lives as we outlined in Chapter 4. Estrogen can be deleterious in certain ways to the type of patient studied in the WHI, with an average age of 63 and with higher cardiovascular risk factors than younger patients. Actually, the higher risk of stroke and thromboembolic disease found in these patients is NOT new information. This is simply corroborative of prior studies done decades ago.

What IS new information is that HT is no longer recommended for primary prevention of cardiovascular disease in the typical WHI patient. Even newer information from 2006 is that now we DO HAVE statistically significant evidence that HT can actually be associated with *lower* heart attack risk and diabetes development in the 50-59 year old group.

The risk of breast cancer increase, even in the older typical WHI patient is miniscule......8 tenths of one percent higher, even if combination estrogen and MPA are utilized. If estrogen alone is utilized, the patient is actually lowering her breast cancer risk compared with taking nothing and just "sweating it out", which is a risk factor in and of itself for Alzheimer's Syndrome. Also, we found out that significant improvement in quality of life is noted in women taking HT between 50- 59. ***All of this is excellent news***.

However, the typical WHI patient is ***not*** truly representative of the type of patients who present to us for symptomatic menopausal evaluation. We see much younger patients who could benefit selectively from HT, sometimes dramatically so, especially relative to quality of life issues. If they choose to go on HT after verbal informed consent, they should be given it by prescription, carefully monitored, and kept on the lowest dose for the shortest time period, according to current dogma. This may change in the future.

We have also discovered that interpretation of scientific data can be tricky, and that careful reanalysis can give totally different conclusions. For example, it has been argued that the average age of 63 of the WHI patient means that half the patients were younger than this. Yes, but those same 63 year olds become average 68 year olds in 5 years. Should we base the health of a generation of early 50 year old menopausal women on a population of late 60-early seventy somethings? No. Should we treat a 32 year old patient with onset of severe menopausal symptoms after ovarian removal the same as we treat a 70 year old? I think not. One size does not fit all and medicine is not that simple.

In summary, we do feel the WHI has been a milestone of medical investigation. As physicians, we are much more careful in menopausal evaluation, and in the monitoring of HT in our patients. Patients, in turn, have become much more inquisitive, and read voraciously. We have seen that medical decision making can be totally turned upside down by premature interpretation of raw data and release by non-practicing clinicians.

We have also witnessed what happens when a confused media is allowed to cry wolf in a crowded theater in an Internet based world. Kansas tornados take us to the Land of Oz, and we are still trying to slide down the rainbow back home. We have only begun to decipher the hieroglyphics. It is very likely the final chapter about HT will not be deciphered in any of our lifetimes. Stay tuned…the best is yet to come.

ભ ભ ભ

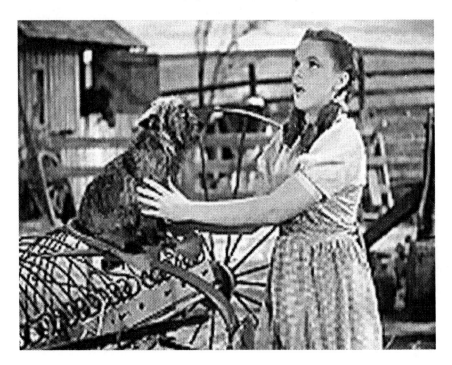

Chapter 18

Women of a Certain Age

by Andy Rooney of CBS's 60 Minutes

As I grow in age, I value women who are over 50 most of all. Here are the reasons why: A woman over 50 will not lie next to you in bed and ask, "What are you thinking?" She doesn't care what you think! If a woman over 50 doesn't want to watch the game, she doesn't sit around whining about it. She does something she wants to do. And it's usually something more interesting? A woman over 50 knows herself well enough to be assured in who she is, what she is, what she wants and from whom.

Few women past the age the age of 50 give a damn what you might think of her or what she is doing? Women over 50 are dignified. They seldom have a screaming match with you at the Opera or in the middle of an expensive restaurant. Of course, if you deserve it, they won't hesitate to shoot you, if they think that they can get away with it! Older women are generous with praise, often undeserved. They know what it's like to be unappreciated. A woman over 50 has the self assurance to introduce you to her woman friends. A younger woman with a man will often ignore even her best friend because she doesn't trust the guy with other women! Women over 50 couldn't care less if you are attracted to her friends because she knows her friends won't betray her? Women get very psychic as they age.

You never have to confess your sins to a woman over 50. They always know! A woman over 50 always looks good wearing bright red lipstick. This is not true of younger women or drag queens.? Once you get past a wrinkle or two, a woman over 50 is far sexier than her younger counterpart? Older women are forthright and honest. They will tell you right off if you are a jerk or if you are acting like one! You don't ever have to wonder where you stand with her.?

Yes, we praise women over 50 for a multitude of reasons. Unfortunately, it's not reciprocal. For every stunning, smart, well coiffed hot woman of 50+, there is a bald, paunchy relic in bright yellow pants making a fool of himself with some 18 year old waitress,? Ladies, I apologize? For all those men who say, "Why buy the cow when you can get the milk free?" Here's an update for you! Nowadays 80% of women are against marriage, why? Because women realize it's not worth buying an entire Pig, just to get a little sausage!

Recommended Reading List

1) Avis, et al., Psychosocial, Behavioral, and Health Factors Related To Menopausal Symptomatology. Womens Health 1997; 3:103-120.

2) A Woman's Guide to Menopause and Perimenopause, by Mary Jane Minkin, M.D., and Carol V. Wright, Ph.D., Yale University Press Health and Wellness, 2005.

3) Berman, BM, et. al., The Public Debate Over Alternative Medicine: The Importance of Finding a Middle Ground. Alter Ther Health Med 2000; 6:98-101.

4) Body and Soul Magazine, Watertown, Massachusetts.

5) Bone Density: (JAMA, 290: No.1, October 13, 2003)

6) Breast Cancer: (JAMA, 289: No. 24, June 25, 2003)

7) Buckler, H. M. et. al. Which Androgen Replacement Therapy For Women? J Clin Endocrinol Metab. 1998; 83: 3920-3924.

8) Buckman, R. and Lewith, G. What Does Homeopathy Do----and how? BMJ 1994; 309: 103-106.

9) Colorectal Cancer: (NEJM, Vol. 350: p. 991-1004, March 4, 2004)

10) Cognitive Function: (JAMA, 289: No. 20. May 28, 2003)

11) Diabetes: (Diabetologia, July, 2004)

12) Espeland, M.A. et al. for the Womens Health Initiative Memory Study Investigators. Conjugated Equine Estrogens and Global Cognitive Function in Postmenopausal Function: WHIMS. JAMA 2004; 291: 2959-2968.

13) Fit For Life, By Dr. Edward Taub, First Edition, McGraw-Hill Publishers, New York, NY, 2001.

14) Fugh-Berman, Adriane and Kronenberg, Fredi. Herbs Used For Menopausal Symptoms, Vol. 4, No. 9, p. 65-72, September 2003.

15) Griebling, T.L. and Nygaard, I.E. The Role Of Estrogen Replacement Therapy in The Management of Urinary Incontinence and Urinary Tract Infection in Post-Menopausal Women. Endocrinol Metab Clin North Amer 1997; 26: 347-360.

16) Greenblatt, R.B. et.al., Evaluation of an Estrogen, Androgen, Estrogen-Androgen Combination, and a Placebo in The Treatment of Menopause. J. Clinical Endocrinology Metabolism. 1950; 10: 1547-1558.

17) Greendale, G.A., et. al., Late Physical and Functional Effects of Osteoporotic Fractures in Women: The Rancho Bernado Study. J. Am Geriatr Soc 1995; 43: 955-961.

18) Grodstein, et al. Postmenopausal Hormone Therapy and Cognitive Function in Healthy Older Women. J Am Geriatr Soc 2000; 48: 746-752.

19) Grodstein, F. , Manson, J.E., and Stampfer, M.J. Hormone Therapy and Coronary Heart Disease: The Role of Time Since Menopause and Age at Hormone Initiation. J. Womens Health (Larchmt); 200615:35-44.

20) Heart Disease: (NEJM, 349: 523-534, August 7, 2003) and 37) Archives of Internal Medicine, 166: No. 3, February 13, 2006).

21) Henderson, V.W., The Epidemiology of Estrogen Replacement Therapy and Alzheimer's Disease. Neurology. 1997; 48(5 Suppl 7): 527-535.

22) Hormone Balance Eating, First Edition, by Robert A. Greene M.D.

23) Hsia, et. al., Conjugated Equine Estrogens and Coronary Heart Disease: The Women's Health Initiative. Arch. Internal Medicine. 2006; 166:357-365.

24) Karas, Richard H., Post-Menopausal Hormone Therapy and Coronary Heart Disease: Is There A Critical Time Period To Produce Benefit? Council on Hormone Education, Volume 4, No.1., 1-9.

25) Kritz-Silverstein, D., et al., Isoflavones and Cognitive Function in Older Women: The Soy and Postmenopausal Health in Aging (SOPHIA) Study. Menopause. 2003; 10:196-202.

26) Kronenberg, F. Hot Flashes. In Lobo, R.A., Ed. Treatment of The Post-Menopausal Woman : Basic and Clinical Aspects. Second Edition. Philadelphia , PA. : Lippencott Williams and Wilkins; 1999:157-177.

27) Laumann, E.O., et al. Sexual Dysfunction in the United States: Prevalence and Predictors. JAMA 1999; 281:537-544.

28) Loving What Is, First Edition, by Byron Katie, Three Rivers Press, N.Y. 2002.

29) Lung Cancer: (Cancer Research, University of Pittsburgh Cancer Institute Publication, February 15, 2005)

30) MacEoin, B., Homeopathy For Menopause. Rochester, VT: Healing Arts Press; 1997.

31) Management of Osteoporosis in Postmenopausal Women: Position Statement: Osteoporosis, NAMS. Menopause 2006; 3: 340-367.

32) Meils, G.B., et al., Ipriflavone Prevents Bone Loss in Postmenopausal Women. Menopause. 1996; 3: 27-32.

33) Menopause Practice: A Clinician's Guide. 2004. Published by the The North American Menopause Society, ISBN 0-9701251-6-X.

34) Murkes, A. et al., Phytoestrogens and Breast Cancer in Postmenopausal Women: A Case-Control Study. Menopause. 2000; 7: 289-296.

35) Natchtigall, L.E., et al., Serum Estradiol-Binding Profiles in Post-Menopausal Women Undergoing Three Common Estrogen Replacement Therapies: Associations With Sex Hormone Binding Globulin.

36) National Institutes of Health Office of Altrenative Medicine, Practice and Policy Guidelines. Clinical Practice Guidelines in Complimentary and Alternative Medicinc: An Analysis of Opportunities and Obstacles. Arch Fam Med 1997; 6: 149-154.

37) National Osteoporosis Foundation. Physician's Guide To Prevention and Treatment of Osteoporosis. Washington, D.C. National Osteoporosis Foundation.; 2003.

38) Osmers, R., et al., Efficacy and Safety of Isopropanolic Black Cohosh Extract for Climacteric Symptoms. Obstetrics and Gynecology, 2005:1074-1083.

39) Other Gynecologic Malignancies: (JAMA: 290: No. 13, October 1, 2003)

40) Peganini-Hill, A. and Henderson, V.W. Estrogen Replacement Therapy and Risk of Alzheimer's Disease. Arch Inter Med . 1996; 156:2213-2217.

41) Practical Guide to Diagnosing and Managing HSDD in Post-Menopausal Women, Advanstar Medical Economics Healthcare Education, 2005.

42) <u>Quality of Life</u>: (NEJM, May 18, 2003) and (JAMA, 294: No. 2, July 13, 2005)

43) Recommendations for Estrogen and Progestogen Use In Peri- and Post-Menopausal Women: October 2004 Position Statement NAMS. Menopause 2004; 11: 589-600.

44) Reddy, S.Y. et al., Gabapentin, Estrogen, and Placebo for Treating Hot Flashes: A Randomized Controlled Trial. Obstetrics and Gynecology. 2006: 108: No. 1, 41-48.

45) Sarrel, Phil M. , Sexuality and Menopause. Obstetrics and Gynecology. 1990; 75: 26S-30S.

46) Sarrel, Phil M., et al., Estrogen and Estrogen-Androgen Replacement In Post-Menopausal Women Dissatisfied With Estrogen Only Therapy. J. Reproductive Med 1998;43: 847-856.

47) Schumaker, S.A., Legault, C. , Kuller, L., et. al. Conjugated Equine Estrogens and the Incidence of Probable Dementia and Mild Cognitive Impairment in Post-Menopausal Women: Womens Health Initiative Memory Study . JAMA. 2004: 291: 3005-3007.

48) Sherwin, B.B., Estrogen and Cognitive Function in Women. Endocr Rev 2003; 24:133-151.

49) Speroff, Leon, Menopause: A Clinician's Guidebook. Guidelines for Contemporary Management. 2005 Advanstar Communications.

50) <u>Stroke</u>: (JAMA, 289: No. 20, May 28, 2003)

51) The Role Of Isoflavones in Menopausal Health: Consensus Opinion, NAMS. Menopause 2000; 7: 215-229.

52) The Role of Testosterone Therapy in Menopausal Women: Position Statement, NAMS. Menopause 2005; 12: 497-511.

53) The Sexy Years, First Edition, by Suzanne Somers and Robert A. Greene, M.D. Crown Publishers, N.Y. 2004.

54) The Women's Health Initiative Study, Journal of the American Medical Association: 288: 321-333, 2002.

55) Think Positive Thoughts Every Day Special Edition by Patricia Wayant, Blue Mountain Press Boulder, Colorado 2003.

56) Treatment of Menopause-Associated Vasomotor Symptoms: Position Statement, NAMS. Menopause 2004; 11: 11-13.

57) <u>Urinary Incontinence</u>: (JAMA, 293: No. 8, February 23, 2005)

58) <u>Venous Thrombosis</u>: (JAMA, 292: No. 13, October 6, 2004)

59) <u>Vitamin D and Calcium Supplementation</u>: (NEJM: 354:669-683, February 16, 2006)

60) Wrinkle Free Forever, First Edition, by Dr. Howard Murad, M.D., St. Martins Griffen, N.Y. 2003.

Informational Resources for MJTFM

- American Association of Clinical Endocrinologists: **www.aace.com**

- American Cancer Society: **www.cancer.org**

- American College of Obstetricians and Gynecologists: **www.acog.org**

- American Heart Association: **www.americanheart.org**

- American Lung Association: **www.lungusa.org**

- Menopause Just The Facts, Ma'am: **www.justthefactsmaam.net**

- National Cancer Institute: **www.nci.nih.gov**

- National Center for Complimentary and Alternative Medicine: **www.nccam.nih.gov**

- National Library of Medicine: **www.nlm.nih.gov**

- National Heart, Lung, and Blood Institute: **www.nhlbi.nih.gov**

- National Osteoporosis Foundation: **www.nof.org**

- National Women's Health Network: **www.womenshealthnetwork.org**

- North American Menopause Society: **www.menopause.org**

- The Hormone Foundation: **www.hormone.org**

- The Women's Health Initiative: **www.whi.org**

- Wyeth Educational: **www.knowmenopause.com**

Printed in the United States
58799LVS00004BA/1-24